AF294346

ATLAS OF SELECTIVE SENTINEL LYMPHADENECTOMY FOR MELANOMA, BREAST CANCER AND COLON CANCER

Cancer Treatment and Research

Steven T. Rosen, M.D., *Series Editor*

Goldstein, L.J., Ozols, R. F. (eds.): *Anticancer Drug Resistance. Advances in Molecular and Clinical Research.* 1994. ISBN 0-7923-2836-1.

Hong, W.K., Weber, R.S. (eds.): *Head and Neck Cancer. Basic and Clinical Aspects.* 1994. ISBN 0-7923-3015-3.

Thall, P.F. (ed): *Recent Advances in Clinical Trial Design and Analysis.* 1995. ISBN 0-7923-3235-0.

Buckner, C. D. (ed): *Technical and Biological Components of Marrow Transplantation.* 1995. ISBN 0-7923-3394-2.

Winter, J.N. (ed.): *Blood Stem Cell Transplantation.* 1997. ISBN 0-7923-4260-7.

Muggia, F.M. (ed): *Concepts, Mechanisms, and New Targets for Chemotherapy.* 1995. ISBN 0-7923-3525-2.

Klastersky, J. (ed): *Infectious Complications of Cancer.* 1995. ISBN 0-7923-3598-8.

Kurzrock, R., Talpaz, M. (eds): *Cytokines: Interleukins and Their Receptors.* 1995. ISBN 0-7923-3636-4.

Sugarbaker, P. (ed): *Peritoneal Carcinomatosis: Drugs and Diseases.* 1995. ISBN 0-7923-3726-3.

Sugarbaker, P. (ed): *Peritoneal Carcinomatosis: Principles of Management.* 1995. ISBN 0-7923-3727-1.

Dickson, R.B., Lippman, M.E. (eds.): *Mammary Tumor Cell Cycle, Differentiation and Metastasis.* 1995. ISBN 0-7923-3905-3.

Freireich, E.J, Kantarjian, H. (eds.): *Molecular Genetics and Therapy of Leukemia.* 1995. ISBN 0-7923-3912-6.

Cabanillas, F., Rodriguez, M.A. (eds.): *Advances in Lymphoma Research.* 1996. ISBN 0-7923-3929-0.

Miller, A.B. (ed.): *Advances in Cancer Screening.* 1996. ISBN 0-7923-4019-1.

Hait , W.N. (ed.): *Drug Resistance.* 1996. ISBN 0-7923-4022-1.

Pienta, K.J. (ed.): *Diagnosis and Treatment of Genitourinary Malignancies.* 1996. ISBN 0-7923-4164-3.

Arnold, A.J. (ed.): *Endocrine Neoplasms.* 1997. ISBN 0-7923-4354-9.

Pollock, R.E. (ed.): *Surgical Oncology.* 1997. ISBN 0-7923-9900-5.

Verweij, J., Pinedo, H.M., Suit, H.D. (eds.): *Soft Tissue Sarcomas: Present Achievements and Future Prospects.* 1997. ISBN 0-7923-9913-7.

Walterhouse, D.O., Cohn, S. L. (eds.): *Diagnostic and Therapeutic Advances in Pediatric Oncology.* 1997. ISBN 0-7923-9978-1.

Mittal, B.B., Purdy, J.A., Ang, K.K. (eds.): *Radiation Therapy.* 1998. ISBN 0-7923-9981-1.

Foon, K.A., Muss, H.B. (eds.): *Biological and Hormonal Therapies of Cancer.* 1998. ISBN 0-7923-9997-8.

Ozols, R.F. (ed.): *Gynecologic Oncology.* 1998. ISBN 0-7923-8070-3.

Noskin, G. A. (ed.): *Management of Infectious Complications in Cancer Patients.* 1998. ISBN 0-7923-8150-5

Bennett, C. L. (ed.): *Cancer Policy.* 1998. ISBN 0-7923-8203-X

Benson, A. B. (ed.): *Gastrointestinal Oncology.* 1998. ISBN 0-7923-8205-6

Tallman, M.S. , Gordon, L.I. (eds.): *Diagnostic and Therapeutic Advances in Hematologic Malignancies.* 1998. ISBN 0-7923-8206-4

von Gunten, C.F. (ed.): *Palliative Care and Rehabilitation of Cancer Patients.* 1999. ISBN 0-7923-8525-X

Burt, R.K., Brush, M.M. (eds): *Advances in Allogeneic Hematopoietic Stem Cell Transplantation.* 1999. ISBN 0-7923-7714-1

Angelos, P. (ed): *Ethical Issues in Cancer Patient Care* 2000. ISBN 0-7923-7726-5

Gradishar, W.J., Wood, W.C. (eds): *Advances in Breast Cancer Management.* 2000. ISBN 0-7923-7890-3

Sparano, Joseph A. (ed.): *HIV & HTLV-I Associated Malignancies.* 2001. ISBN 0-7923-7220-4.

Ettinger, David S. (ed.): *Thoracic Oncology.* 2001. ISBN 0-7923-7248-4.

Bergan, Raymond C. (ed.): *Cancer Chemoprevention.* 2001. ISBN 0-7923-7259-X.

Raza, A., Mundle, S.D. (eds): *Myelodysplastic Syndromes & Secondary Acute Myelogenous Leukemia* 2001. 0-7923-7396-0.

Talamonti, Mark S. (ed.): *Liver Directed Therapy for Primary and Metastatic Liver Tumors.* 2001. ISBN 0-7923-7523-8.

Stack, M.S., Fishman, D.A. (eds): *Ovarian Cancer.* 2001. ISBN 0-7923-7530-0.

Bashey, A., Ball, E.D. (eds): *Non-Myeloablative Allogeneic Transplantation.* 2002. ISBN 0-7923-7646-3

ATLAS OF SELECTIVE SENTINEL LYMPHADENECTOMY FOR MELANOMA, BREAST CANCER AND COLON CANCER

edited by

Stanley P.L. Leong
University of California, San Francisco, U.S.A.

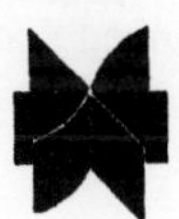

SPRINGER SCIENCE+BUSINESS MEDIA, LLC

ISBN 978-1-4757-7631-7   ISBN 978-0-306-47822-2 (eBook)
DOI 10.1007/978-0-306-47822-2

Library of Congress Cataloging-in-Publication Data

A C.I.P. Catalogue record for this book is available
from the Library of Congress.

*The Publisher offers discounts on this book for course use and bulk purchases.
For further information, send email to laura.walsh@wkap.com.*

TABLE OF CONTENTS

PREFACE vi

ACKNOWLEDGEMENTS vii

CONTRIBUTORS viii

CHAPTER 1   *Rationale and Development of Sentinel Lymph Node Dissection*
Jan H. Wong, MD 1

CHAPTER 2   *Lymphoscintigraphy in the Detection of Sentinel Lymph Nodes*
Eugene T. Morita, MD 9

CHAPTER 3   *Selective Sentinel Lymph Node Mapping and Dissection for Malignant Melanoma*
Stanley P. L. Leong, MD 39

CHAPTER 4   *Selective Sentinel Lymph Node Mapping and Dissection for Breast Cancer*
Stanley P. L. Leong, MD 65

CHAPTER 5   *Pathologic Examination of the Sentinel Lymph Node*
Patrick A. Treseler, PhD 81

CHAPTER 6   *Selective Lymph Node Mapping in Colorectal Cancer – A Prospective Study for Impact on Staging, Limitations and Pitfalls*
Sukamal Saha, MD 109

SELECTED READINGS 117

INDEX 119

PREFACE

The underlying thesis in solid cancer biology is that metastasis in general starts in an orderly progression with lymphatic spread first to the sentinel lymph node (SLN) in the nearest lymph node basin. Therefore, the logical approach is to harvest that specific SLN for thorough analysis. Because a tumor-free SLN is usually associated with a negative residual lymph node basin, a negative SLN is an excellent indication that micrometastasis has not occurred in the regional lymph nodes. When the SLN is involved it is not known whether or not metastasis is limited only to the SLN or if the disease has spread to the remainder of the nodal basin. For this reason, if a SLN is positive, a complete lymph node dissection is indicated. Thus, a selective sentinel lymphadenectomy should be considered as a staging procedure so that patients with negative SLNs (about 80%) may be spared an extended lymph node dissection.

Malignant melanoma has been proven to be the most ideal tumor model to study the role of SLN. Subsequently, selective sentinel lymphadenectomy has been applied to breast cancer, colon cancer and other types of solid cancer. The multidisciplinary approach encompassing the surgeon, nuclear medicine physician, and pathologist is the key to such a successful procedure. Beyond the technical aspects of harvesting the SLN, the implication of micrometastasis remains to be defined. Follow-up of patients after selective sentinel lymphadenectomy is crucial.

Since selective sentinel lymphadenectomy is a recently developed technique, most surgeons who are actively practicing surgery have not learned this procedure during their formal training years. Therefore, it is important for the surgeons to learn this technique through well designed lymphatic mapping courses and observe actual operative procedures of selective sentinel lymphadenectomy to achieve proficiency. It is imperative that the surgeon should learn this technique properly so that the most accurate SLN may be harvested. Thus, it is timely to have a book entirely dedicated to the theory and practice of selective sentinel lymphadenectomy combining preoperative and interoperative lymphatic mapping approaches. Further, evaluation of the SLN requires meticulous assessment of the SLN with multiple sections and immunohistochemistry.

This atlas is tailored to bring the practical aspects of selective sentinel lymphadenectomy for melanoma, breast and colon cancer into focus so that practitioners can use it as a reference manual. It is important to emphasize the multidisciplinary approach of harvesting SLN(s) incorporating the experiences of a nuclear medicine physician, a surgeon, and a pathologist. Such a team can be formed readily with appropriate training.

Stanley P. L. Leong, MD

Department of Surgery
UCSF Comprehensive Cancer Center
1600 Divisadero Street
San Francisco, California 94115

ACKNOWLEDGEMENTS

This work was supported in part by a grant from the Eva B. Buck Charitable Trust; William S. Graham Foundation for Melanoma Research, Inc., Castro Valley, CA (www.bfmelanoma.com); Neoprobe Corporation, Dublin, Ohio; Schering Biotech Oncology, Kenilworth, NJ; Immunex, Seattle, WA; Becton-Dickinson, San Jose, CA; Dendreon, Seattle, WA; and Ethicon Endo-Surgery, Inc., Cincinnati, Ohio.

We appreciate the excellent work of Rachel Seaman and Emily Huang in the preparation of this book. We also appreciate the excellent graphics work of Jean Chan, UCSF Graphic Arts Department.

CONTRIBUTORS

Stanley P. L. Leong, MD, Professor, and Director, Sentinel Lymph Node Program, Department of Surgery, University of California, San Francisco Medical Center at Mount Zion; and Member, UCSF Comprehensive Cancer Center, San Francisco, California

Eugene T. Morita, MD, Clinical Professor of Nuclear Medicine and Radiology, and Chief, Section of Nuclear Medicine, Department of Radiology, University of California, San Francisco/Mount Zion Medical Center, San Francisco, California

Sukamal Saha, MD, FRCS(C), Assistant Professor of Surgery and Anatomy, Michiagan State University College of Human Medicine; and the Department of Surgery, McLaren Regional Medical Center, Flint, Michigan

Patrick A. Treseler, MD, PhD, Associate Director of Surgical Pathology and Clinical Professor of Pathology, Department of Pathology, University of California, San Francisco

Jan H. Wong, MD, Professor, Department of Surgery, University of Hawaii John A. Burns School of Medicine, Honolulu, Hawaii

1 RATIONALE AND DEVELOPMENT OF SENTINEL LYMPH NODE DISSECTION

Jan H. Wong, MD

INTRODUCTION

One of the longest standing and most controversial issues in the management of the patient with cutaneous melanoma has been the therapeutic value of immediate lymphadenectomy in the clinically node-negative individual. In 1892, Herbert Snow [1892] noted that "the danger lies in the diffusion of malignant cells….These always implicate the nearest lymph glands….Palpable enlargement of these gland is, unfortunately, but a late symptom of deposits therein….We see the paramount importance of securing the perfect eradication of these lymph glands which will necessarily be first infected." Numerous single institutional reports have suggested improved survival in patients who undergo immediate lymphadenectomy when compared with individuals who undergo lymphadenectomy for clinically evident disease [Balch 1981, Koh 1986, Morton 1991, Roses 1985, Callery 1982]. These reports, however, have been criticized because of their retrospective nature and the utilization of historical controls. In contrast, three prospective randomized trials have failed to confirm the survival advantage noted in these single institutional retrospective analyses [Balch 1996, Sim 1986, Veronesi 1977] and raised the possibility that regional nodal metastases might be an indicator of systemic disease rather than a marker of the orderly progression of disease from the primary tumor. As a result of the World Health Organization Trial [Veronesi 1977, 1982] the standard of care in the management of apparently localized cutaneous melanoma has been considered wide excision of the primary site and observation.

Although a number of alternative explanations to explain the lack of benefit observed in these prospective randomized trials were proposed, perhaps the most compelling reason for failing to demonstrate any statistically significant improvement in survival was the inability to accurately stage patients. It is apparent that only those individuals with pathologically involved nodes *and* without metastatic disease were the only individuals that could potentially benefit from immediate node dissection. The majority of patients either did not have nodal metastases or nodal metastases were associated with non-regional micrometastatic disease. These individuals, therefore, could not even, theoretically, benefit from an immediate lymphadenectomy. Natural history studies suggests that individuals who are node positive but without non-regional micrometastatic disease represented only a small minority of the patients studied in these prospective, randomized trials and raised the possibility that that these trials might not have had sufficient statistical power to identify a survival advantage. Additionally, the Intergroup Melanoma Surgical Program Trial [Balch 1996] was several years away from completion and analysis.

Because of the possibility that earlier trials did not have the statistical power to identify survival advantage, we initiated studies at the University of California, Los Angeles to determine whether operative approaches could be developed to identify node metastases in clinically node negative individuals who could potentially benefit from immediate lymphadenectomy while sparing the majority of node negative individuals the morbidity of complete node dissection that would have no potential therapeutic benefit.

SENTINEL NODE CONCEPT AND INTRAOPERATIVE LYMPHATIC MAPPING

In 1977, Cabanas [1977] reported on a novel approach to staging carcinoma of the penis. This new approach was based upon the hypothesis that if carcinoma of the penis metastasized, it would do so to a node that was located medially and superiorly to the saphenofemoral junction in each groin. Cabanas developed this hypothesis after extensive anatomic studies using lymphangiograms to determine the lymphatic anatomy of the penis in 100 patients. Cabanas coined the term *sentinel node* to describe this node and suggested that if the sentinel node was found to have metastatic disease, the patient required a formal lymphadenectomy. Conversely, when the sentinel node was found to be free of metastatic disease, the likelihood of identifying metastatic disease in the groin was low and no further resection was necessary.

The concept that a primary solid tumor would preferentially drain through the lymphatics to a *specific* a lymph node and that the status of that lymph node would reflect the histology of the regional lymphatic basin was revolutionary. Independently of Cabanas, in the mid 1980's, we, at the University of California, Los Angeles similarly proposed that the lymphatic drainage of a primary tumor would be to a specific lymph node [Wong 1991]. In contrast to Cabanas, however, we believed that the lymphatic drainage might vary from patient to patient and not necessarily in a fixed anatomic location. Therefore, to reproducibly identify the sentinel node, intraoperative techniques would need to be developed to define the lymphatic drainage of a given primary tumor site rather than utilize an operative approach that was dependent upon the anatomy.

FELINE STUDIES

At the time of our original work, the relationship between the skin, dermal lymphatics and regional lymph nodes was poorly understood. Classical anatomic studies by Sappey [1874] had suggested a relatively narrow strip of skin with ambiguous lymphatic drainage about the level of the umbilicus and in the midline. However, physiologic studies utilizing radiocolloids suggests substantially more variability in the lymphatic drainage of the skin [Norman 1991]. We hypothesized that despite the complexity of the dermal lymphatic, a particular area of skin would drain to a single, sentinel, lymph node. In order to test this hypothesis, we investigated a number of potential animal models that might mimic the regional lymphatics of the human [Wong 1991]. However, most animals have a single large node in the superficial node basin and were not appropriate to test the sentinel lymph node hypothesis. However, the cat has three separate lymph nodes in the groin, somewhat analogous to the anatomy of humans and this was the animal model utilized to further develop operative approaches to identifying the sentinel lymph node.

A number of agents were examined to determine the feasibility of intraoperative identification of the sentinel lymph node. The vital blue dye, isosulfan blue, proved to be the most useful agent to map the dermal lymphatics. Following the intradermal injection of isosulfan blue, an incision was made in the inguinal crease and skin flaps were elevated. The inguinal fat pad was resected and carefully oriented. The lymph nodes were then examined for the presence or absence of blue stained lymph nodes. Rapid uptake of isosulfan blue was observed and allowed for ready visualization of the lymphatic channels and lymph nodes that were stained blue.

These studies demonstrated that the intradermal injection of a lymphatic dye, isosulfan blue, resulted in the rapid uptake of the dye in the dermal lymphatics and that with meticulous dissection, these dermal lymphatics could be followed to a regional lymph node. The skin of the hind limb, abdomen, and perineum were all used as sites of injection and the specific lymph node that was stained blue was determined. A predictable pattern of lymphatic drainage emerged from the various anatomic sites of injection. Each skin sites would drain only to a specific lymph node and there appeared to be well-defined borders between different areas of skin that would drain to the medial, middle or lateral inguinal node of the cat. These results clearly supported the concept of a sentinel lymph node and the feasibility of an intraoperative approach to identifying the lymphatic drainage of specific skin site. This operative procedure was termed *selective lymphadenectomy*.

PATIENT INVESTIGATION IN CUTANEOUS MELANOMA

Based upon the hypothesis that operative techniques, developed to identify the dermal lymphatic drainage in a feline model, could be used to identify lymph node that would be the primary drainage of cutaneous melanoma, we began patient investigations at UCLA. The operative technique of intraoperative lymphatic mapping and selective lymphadenectomy evolved from a blunt blind dissection to identify blue-stained lymph nodes to a very refined operative technique. Cutaneous lymphoscintigraphy was utilized to identify lymphatic drainage in areas of ambiguous lymphatic drainage such as the trunk and skin of the head and neck. The patients were then taken to the operating room where isosulfan blue was injected intradermally. Injections were repeated every 20 minutes. The injection site was gently massaged and an incision in the anticipated site of the sentinel lymph node was made. As in the feline model, careful elevation of skin flaps was performed and utilizing a blunt dissection technique, blue stained lymph nodes were searched for prior to performing an immediate completion node dissection.

The initial operative technique evolved toward careful dissection in the area of the presumed afferent lymphatic channel, which was stained blue by the isosulfan blue. Once identified, the blue stained lymphatic channel would be followed meticulously through the regional nodal fat basin, and if the lymphatic channel was not disrupted, to a blue stained lymph node. This blue stained node was characterized as the "sentinel" lymph node. Following completion of the selective lymphadenectomy, a formal regional node dissection was performed.

Two hundred thirty three consecutive patients undergoing surgical management of their primary cutaneous melanoma were studied. Successful identification of a blue stained lymph node occurred in 82% of cases. Forty-eight lymphadenectomy specimens were found to have metastatic tumor. All but two of these lymphadenectomy specimens had tumor present in the blue stained lymph node [Morton 1992]. The false negative rate of approximately 5% has subsequently been substantiated by a number of other institutions [Gershenwald 1999, Leong 1997, Reintgen 1994, Ross 1993, Wong 2000].

As originally described, selective lymphadenectomy was an intraoperative technique that required substantial experience to master. In 1977, cutaneous lymphoscintigraphy was introduced to define the lymphatic drainage of ambiguous skin sites [Holmes 1977]. Because of the variability in the location of the sentinel lymph node, harvesting the sentinel lymph node often times required a more extensive dissection than was intended. Employing cutaneous lymphoscintigraphy, the general location within the regional lymphatic basin could be identified. Dermal markings were employed to help minimize the extent of the surgical procedure [Reintgen 1994]. However, it was development of hand held gamma probes that had been developed and investigated in radioimmunoguided surgery that has led to broad application of selective lymphadenectomy.

RADIOGUIDED SELECTIVE LYMPHADENECTOMY

In 1993, Alex and Krag reported on the use of a hand held gamma probe to identify regional nodes that taken up technetium labeled sulfur colloid [Alex 1993]. Because of the technical difficulty of intraoperative lymphatic mapping and the prolonged learning curves to acquire satisfactory outcomes [Morton 1992, 1997], radioguided techniques provided a much simpler technique to identify and harvest the sentinel lymph node while minimizing the extent of the surgical dissection. It has not been confirmed that whether a radioguided technique [Krag 1995], a isosulfan blue directed dissection [Morton 1992, Thompson 1995] or a combination of the two techniques [Wong 2000, Albertini 1996a, Essner 2000] that harvesting of the sentinel node accurately reflects the histology of the regional lymphatic basin in cutaneous melanoma.

SELECTIVE LYMPHADENECTOMY IN BREAST CANCER

In contrast to cutaneous melanoma in which regional node dissection has historically been considered a potentially therapeutic intervention, axillary node dissection has long been considered an indicator of but not a determinant of outcome [Fisher 1985]. The presence or absence of axillary lymph node metastases remains the most important prognostic factor in apparently localized breast cancer and has been the primary indication for adjuvant systemic therapy. Noninvasive staging of the axilla is inadequate as is physical examination. Based upon the demonstrated accuracy in cutaneous melanoma, Guiliano and coworkers [Giuliano 1994] described the intraoperative technique of sentinel lymphadenectomy for breast cancer in 1994. Like the initial experience in cutaneous melanoma that was pioneered by workers in the same institution [Morton 1992], sentinel lymphadenectomy in breast cancer proved to be technically challenging.

Like the experience in cutaneous melanoma, however, the accuracy of staging the axilla was similar with a false negative rate of 4.3%. And like melanoma, the evolution toward a radioguided approach has resulted in improved harvesting of the sentinel node [Albertini 1996b]. These false negative results have since been duplicated by numerous investigators [Albertini 1996b, Barnwell 1998, Borgstein 1998, Chu 1999, Cody 1999a, Cody 1999b, Cox 1998, Flett 1998, Guenther 1997, Krag 1998, Krag 1993, Offodile 1998], indicating that the sentinel lymph node accurately reflects the histology of the regional lymphatic basin.

CONCLUSION

Little doubt exists as to the validity of the sentinel node hypothesis. When melanoma and breast cancer metastasizes to lymph nodes, it does so in a non-random fashion and the node or nodes at greatest risk for harboring metastatic disease can be identified by operative techniques originally demonstrated to be feasible in a feline model and subsequently proven to be useful in patients. The search for an operative technique to identify cutaneous melanoma patients who could potential benefit from a therapeutic lymphadenectomy, while sparing the vast majority of individuals who are node negative the morbidity of that procedure has revolutionized the surgical approach to cutaneous melanoma and breast cancer and hold promise to further refine our understanding of the biology of not only of these two disease but solid neoplasms in general.

REFERENCES

Albertini JJ, Cruse CW, Rapaport D, et al. Intraoperative radiolymphoscintigraphy improves sentinel lymph node identification for patients with melanoma. Annals of Surgery 1996a;223(2):217-224

Albertini JJ, Lyman GH, Cox C, et al. Lymphatic mapping and sentinel node biopsy in the patient with breast cancer. Journal of the American Medical Association 1996b;276(22):1818-1822

Alex J, Weaver D, Fairbank J, Krag D. Gamma-probe-guided lymph node localization in malignant melanoma. Surgical Oncology 1993;2:303-308

Balch CM, Soong S-J, Bartolucci AA, et al. Efficacy of an elective regional lymph node dissection of 1 to 4 mm thick melanomas for patients 60 years of age and younger. Annals of Surgery 1996;224(3):255-266

Balch CM, Soong S-J, Murad TM, et al. A multifactorial analysis of melanoma III. Prognostic factors in melanoma patients with lymph node metastases (Stage II). Annals of Surgery 1981;193(3):377-388

Barnwell JM, Arredondo MA, Kolmorgen D, et al. Sentinel node biopsy in breast cancer. Annals of Surgical Oncology 1998;5(2):126-130

Borgstein P, Pijpers R, Coumans E, et al. Sentinel lymph node biopsy in breast cancer: guidelines and pitfalls of lymphoscintigraphy and gamma probe detection. Journal American College of Surgeons 1998;186(3):275-283

Cabanas RM. An approach for the treatment of penile carcinoma. Cancer 1977;39(2):456-466

Callery C, Cochran AJ, Roe DJ, al. e. Factors prognostic for survival in patients with malignant melanoma spread to the regional lymph nodes. Annals of Surgery 1982;196:69-75

Chu KU, Turner RR, Hansen NM, et al. Sentinel node metastasis in patients with breast carcinoma accurately predicts immunohistochemnically detectable nonsentinel node metastasis. Annals of Surgical Oncology 1999;6(8):756-761

Cody HS. Sentinel lymph node mapping in breast cancer. Oncology 1999a;13(1):25-33

Cody HS, Hill ADK, Tran KN, et al. Credentialing for breast lymphatic mapping: How many cases are enough? Annals of Surgery 1999b;229(5):723-728

Cox CE, Pendas S, Cox JM, et al. Guidelines for sentinel node biopsy and lymphatic mapping of patients with breast cancer. Annals of Surgery 1998;227(5):645-653

Essner R, Bostick PJ, Glass EC, et al. Standarized probe-directed sentinel node dissection in melanoma. Surgery 2000;127(1):26

Flett M, Going J, Stanton P, Cooke T. Sentinel node localization in patients with breast cancer. British Journal of Surgery 1998;85(7):991-993

Fisher B, Redmond C, Fisher E. Ten-year results of a randomized clinical trial comparing radical mastectomy and total mastectomy with or without radiation. New England Journal of Medicine 1985;312:674-681

Gershenwald JE, Thompson W, Mansfield PF, et al. Multi-institutional melanoma lymphatic mapping experience: The prognostic value of sentinel lymph node status in 612 stage I and II melanoma patients. Journal of Clinical Oncology 1999;17(3):976-983

Giuliano AE, Kirgan DM, Guenther JM, Morton DL. Lymphatic mapping and sentinel lymphadenectomy for breast cancer. Annals of Surgery 1994;220(3):391-401

Guenther JM, Krishnamoorthy M, Tan LR. Sentinel lymphadenectomy for breast cancer in a community managed care setting. Cancer Journal 1997;3(6):336-340

Holmes EC, Moseley HS, Morton DL, et al. A rational approach to the surgical management of melanoma. Annals of Surgery 1977;186(4):481-490

Koh HK, Sober AJ, Day CL Jr., et al. Prognosis of clinical stage I melanoma patients with positive elective regional node dissection. Journal of Clinical Oncology 1986;4(8):1238-1244

Krag D, Weaver D, Ashikaga T, et al. The sentinel node in breast cancer: A multicenter validation study. New England Journal of Medicine 1998;339(14):941-946

Krag DN, Meijer SJ, Weaver DL, et al. Minimal-access surgery for staging of malignant melanoma. Archives of Surgery 1995;130(6):654-658

Krag DN, Weaver DL, Alex JC, Fairbanks JT. Surgical resection and radiolocalization of the sentinel lymph node in breast cancer using a gamma probe. Surgical Oncology 1993;2:335-339

Leong SPL, Steinmetz I, Habib FA, et al. Optimal selective sentinel lymph node dissection in primary malignant melanoma. Archives of Surgery 1997;132(6):666-673

Morton DL. Intraoperative lymphatic mapping and sentinel lymphadenectomy: community standard of care or clinical investigation? [comment] Cancer Journal 1997;3(6):328-30

Morton DL, Duan-Ren W, Wong JH, et al. Technical details of intraoperative lymphatic mapping for early stage melanoma. Archives of Surgery 1992;127(4):392-399

Morton DL, Wanek L, Nizze JA, et al. Improved long-term survival after lymphadenectomy of melanoma metastatic to regional nodes: Analysis of prognostic factors in 1134 patients from the John Wayne Cancer Clinic. Annals of Surgery 1991;214(4):491-501

Norman J, Cruse CW, Espinosa C, et al. Redefinition of cutaneous lymphatic drainage with the use of lymphoscintigraphy for malignant melanoma. American Journal of Surgery 1991;162:432-437

Offodile R, Hoh C, Barsky SH, et al. Minimally invasive breast carcinoma staging using lymphatic mapping with radiolabeled dextran. Cancer 1998;82(9):1704-1708

Reintgen D, Cruse CW, Wells K, et al. The orderly progression of melanoma nodal metastases. Annals of Surgery 1994;220(6):759-767

Roses DF, Provet JA, Harris MN, et al. Prognosis of patients with pathologic stage II cutaneous malignant melanoma. Annals of Surgery 1985;201:103-107

Ross MI, Reintgen D, Balch CM. Selective lymphadenectomy: emerging role for lymphatic mapping and sentinel node biopsy in the management of early stage melanoma. Seminars in Surgical Oncology 1993;9(1):219-223

Sappey M. Anatomie, physiologie, pathologie, des vaisseaux lymphatiques consideres ches l'homme et les vertebres. Paris, 1874.

Sim FH, Taylor WF, Pritchard DJ, Soule EH. Lymphadenectomy in the management of stage I malignant melanoma: A prospective randomized study. Mayo Clinic Proceedings 1986;61(3):697-705

Snow H. Melanotic cancerous disease. Lancet 1892;2:872

Thompson JF, McCarthy WH, Bosch CM, et al. Sentinel lymph node status as an indicator of the presence of melanoma in the regional lymph nodes. Melanoma Research 1995;5(4):255-260

Veronesi U, Adamus J, Bandiera DC, et al. Delayed regional lymph node dissection in stage I melanoma of the skin of the lower extremities. Cancer 1982;49(11):2420-2430

Veronesi U, Adamus J, Bandiera DC, et al. Inefficacy of immediate node dissection in stage I melanoma of the limbs. New England Journal of Medicine 1977;297:627-630

Wong JH, Steinemann S, Yonehara C, et al. Sentinel node staging for cutaneous melanoma in a university-affiliated community care setting. Annals of Surgical Oncology 2000;7(6):450-455

Wong JH, Cagle LA, Morton DL. Lymphatic drainage of skin to a sentinel lymph node in a feline model. Annals of Surgery 1991;214(5):637-641

2 LYMPHOSCINTIGRAPHY IN THE DETECTION OF SENTINEL LYMPH NODES

Eugene T. Morita, MD

LYMPHOSCINTIGRAPHY

Background

In the 1970's, Ege [1977, 1983] used subcostal injections of radiocolloid to determine the status of the internal mammary chain in patients with carcinoma of the breast. The radiocolloids traveled via lymphatic channels to nodes where fixed macrophages in the reticular endothelial system engulfed the colloid. Her work was the first to utilize lymphoscintigraphy in a large scale for breast cancer evaluation. The internal mammary nodes with tumor showed decreased or absent activity, and at times, diversion of tracer to the contralateral side because of obstructed lymphatics. While this technique has not been used in recent years it marked the advent of lymphoscintigraphy in patients with breast cancer.

More recently, the concept of the sentinel lymph node (SLN) has developed. The SLN is defined as the first metastatic node. Morton and his colleagues [Morton 1992a, 1992b, 1997a, 1997b, 1999a] were the first to use blue dye and later, radiotracers to locate the SLN in patients with malignant melanoma. The Delphian node in thyroid cancer has been noted in textbooks for years [DeGroot 1996, Daniels 1991]. In 1960, Gould [1960] used the term, "sentinel node", as a commonly positioned node in patients with parotid carcinomas. Cabanas [1977] studied 100 patients with radiographic contrast to determine, what he also, independently described as the sentinel node. He makes no mention of the work by Gould in his references. Cabanas found that in patients with penile cancers; the sentinel nodes could be evaluated with contrast lymphangiography. He also found that patients with negative sentinel node biopsies and negative dissections had the best prognoses. Those with a positive sentinel node and no other involved nodes had slightly worse prognoses, while the patients with positive sentinel nodes and additional positive nodes on completions lymph node dissection had the worst prognoses. His work did not receive acceptance. Wong, Cagle and Morton [1991] used blue dye in a cat model to determine its effectiveness in locating the SLN. Cabanas is not mentioned in their original paper. In 1991, Morton [1992b] used lymphoscintigraphy to determine sentinel node activity. Morton and his colleagues are to be acknowledged for developing the concept of the sentinel node. Eventually, radiotracers were used to find the sentinel node. Krag [1995, 1998], Reingten [1997, 1998a, 1998b] and Giuliano [1994] further promulgated the concept. These groups helped develop the sentinel lymphadenectomy as common practice in oncologic surgery in melanoma and breast cancer. The SLN has been defined in patients using blue dye, radioactive colloids, or both.

The early investigators such as Grant [1959], Turner-Warrick [1953] and Vendrell-Torne [1972] were instrumental in developing the pathophysiology of lymphatic drainage of the breast.

THE TECHNICAL ASPECTS OF LYMPHOSCINTIGRAPHY

Radiopharmeceuticals

Historically, the first tracer used for lymphoscintigraphy was radioactive Gold 198 (Au 198) [Kazem 1968]. The study by Vendrell-Torne [1972] showed migration of tracer after intraparenchymal injections to the axillary and internal mammary nodes. The particles of Au 198 were quite small, similar to the particle size of Antimony sulfide colloid [Uren 1995, DeCicco 1997]. In the study by Vendrell-Torne [1972], patients were put into five groups, receiving injections into either one of the four quadrants of the breast or into the periareolar area. Virtually all patients had drainage into the axillary chain, regardless of the site of injection. With an upper inner quadrant injection, 80% of the patients were found to have uptake into nodes of the internal mammary chain. The outer quadrants had less activity entering the internal mammary chain. Even by the poor imaging characteristics of rectilinear scanning, they were able to find intramammary nodes. Rectilinear scanning is no longer used to any extent in Nuclear Medicine.

The agent that is most available in the United States is Technetium99m Sulfur Colloid made by the thiosulfate method [Kowalsky 1987, Eshima 1996, Glass 1998]. Technetium 99m (Tc99m) is the radioactive atom that is used to tag the colloid lymphoscintigraphy. Tc99m is an ideal agent for imaging and counting because of its physical half-life, ease in compounding and relatively low dose to the patient as well as individuals caring for the patient. Its further benefit is that it gives minimal particulate energy from internal conversion electrons of low abundance of 10 %. In the process of decaying, it gives off a gamma photon of 140 keV. Because of relatively smaller amounts of energy absorbed in tissue, radiation to the patient is lower compared to other tracers such as I-131 which has significant more amount of particulate energy. Tc99m has a physical half-life of 6 hours. Tc99m is the most common tracer used in Nuclear Medicine since it can be complexed to a myriad of compounds such radiopharmeceuticals for the heart, bone and kidney. In lymphoscintigraphy, relatively small doses are given in the range of several hundred microcuries to a millicurie. In other studies in Nuclear Medicine, such as the heart studies, typical doses are in the range of 20 to 25 mCis.

Tc99m is made in a vial where H_2S is created with the resultant formation of a large number of different size colloidal sulfur particles. To obtain more uniformly sized particles, the tracer is filtered through a .22-micron filter, which removes particles whose size is larger than 220 nanometers (nm). A direct method of making Tc99m sulfur colloid can be made from using H2S gas. H2S is highly toxic and requires the use of well-ventilated and isolated fume hood. Particles made by this method have particles in the range of those of antimony colloid.

Other tracers that are available in Europe and Australia include Tc99m antimony colloid and Tc99m albumin minicolloid [De Cicco 1997, Uren 1995]. Tc99m mini albumin colloid is no longer available in the United States. Tc99m albumin (not colloidal) is available in the United States and passes through lymphatic channels and lymph node in a dynamic fashion. Tc99m albumin was been used to define nodal basins in preparation for surgery [Tonakie 1999].

INJECTION OF TRACER

General Comments
Placement of an intradermal injection can be difficult because of near vision not being optimum in older physicians in Nuclear Medicine. The use of a magnifying lens worn over the head can be quite helpful. These can be purchased at nominal cost of around twenty dollars. They come in a variety of focal lengths. As previously described, additional gentle bending of the needle makes a difficult injection easier. The bending of the needle permits the needle to be parallel to the skin.

Melanomas
Hair is shaved prior to preparation of the skin. The skin is prepared by cleaning the area with alcohol or iodine solution. If local anesthesia is not given, Tc99m sulfur colloid injection is intensely painful for a few seconds. Direct injection of Lidocaine causes pain (albeit brief) due to the low pH of the material. Buffered Lidocaine causes no discomfort when the local anesthetic is given intradermally. To buffer the Lidocaine, draw 0.9 cc of one percent Lidocaine (without epinephrine) into a tuberculin syringe and then add 0.1 cc of 8.4 % sodium bicarbonate. Smaller volumes may be drawn using the same 9:1 ratio. The injection is given around the lesion in patients who have their tumors still present or around the resection biopsy site. Note that if the patient has had a wide local tumor resection, the location of the sentinel node may have been disrupted by the procedure. The skin is prepared and the above syringe of Lidocaine buffered with bicarbonate is used to infiltrate the area. At the excisional biopsy site, inject a fraction of a cc (.05 to 0.1 cc) of radiocolloid to make a wheal of 5 to 10 mm at four sites. Using the center point of the biopsy site, inject the four sites, avoiding any incisions, scars or indurated areas. The injection site will cover about a 1-inch squared area. We use a 1/2-inch, 30-gauge needle. If necessary, the 30-gauge needle can be bent to give a more optimal position of the needle tip to enter the skin (Figure 1). The plastic hub of the needle can be used to accomplish the task. Before injecting, make sure that the needle is firmly fixed to the syringe. The needle should be translucent through the skin. Four sites around the resection site are infiltrated with a wheal of Lidocaine of about 5 to 10 mm. This usually entails an administration of around .05 to 0.1 cc of Lidocaine per site. A similar volume of Tc99m sulfur colloid, having a concentration of 500 to 1000 uCi in a volume of 0.5 cc. A single syringe is used in making the intradermal injection of tracer. The Tc99m sulfur colloid should have a high concentration so as to provide activity described above. Immediately following the intradermal injection of Lidocaine, the dose is given. To prevent contamination a sheet isolates the area of the injection site. Contamination will occur if the needle is not tightly set or the injection site leaks under pressure. The same hole of the injection of local

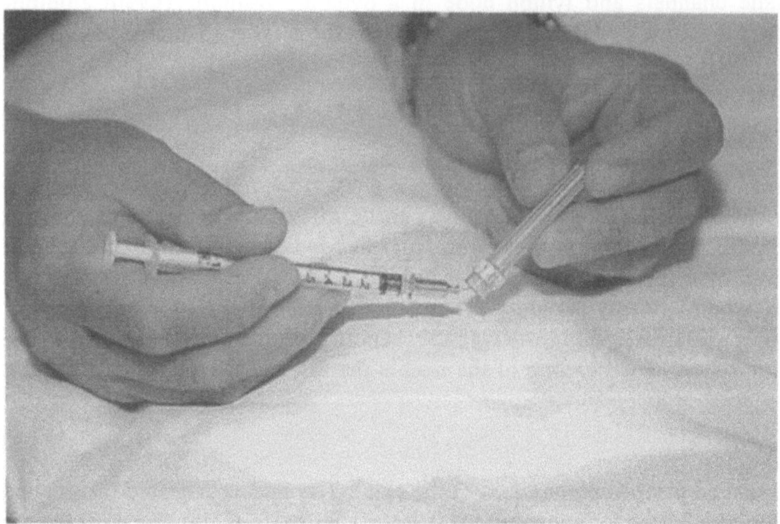

Figure 1. The plastic hub of the needle can be used to bend the needle as noted in the above picture. The bevel of the needle should be placed upward. The needle can be bent in a gentle upward pressure from the plastic needle hub.

anesthesia should be used to inject the colloid. If injected at a different site, leakage from the prior injection site will frequently result. A similar size wheal is given at four sites. After the injection, the area is cleaned with alcohol and then covered with a 2 x 2 inch sterile gauze. The dose given is calculated by subtracting the amount of the residual activity from the initial dose drawn. Imaging begins immediately after the dose is given (Figure 2).

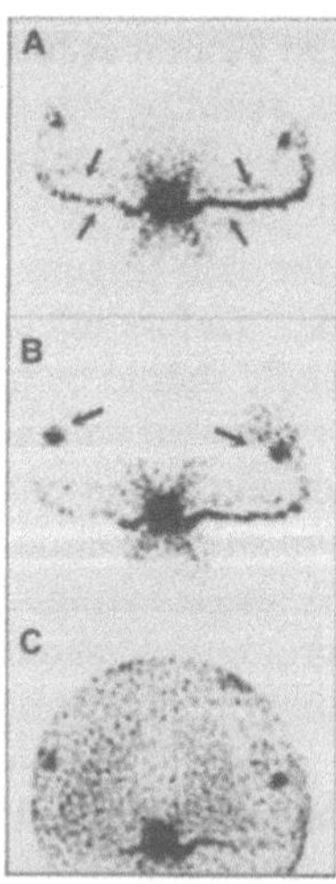

Figure 2. Panel A shows the injection site on the back, the dark area in the center, with two parallel channels (arrows) going into the right and left axillae. Panel B shows the bilateral sentinel nodes (arrows). Panel C is a transmission study of the of the body contours in relationship to the injection site, channels and sentinel lymph nodes.

Special Areas:

I. Toes and Fingers

Generally, three, and occasionally, four sites are injected at the base of the nail. The injection technique described above is used. Generally, local injection at the base of the nail is sufficient to provide good local anesthesia to the toe or finger in patients with subungual melanoma. For patients with larger tumors a nerve block can be accomplished by an anesthetist or surgeon. After anesthesia is obtained, sulfur colloid is injected.

II. Sole of the Foot

The sole of the foot is an extremely difficult area to inject. We ask the anesthesia department to place a local block to the sole of the foot. The patient is asked to arrive about 1 hour before the scheduled time for the study in Nuclear Medicine. Occasionally, the sole is not totally anesthetized and Lidocaine is supplemented. The area is quite bloody when the needle is inserted. Gauze should be readily available. With pain control obtained, the callus of the sole of the foot can be removed. Injecting radiocolloid into a callus will show no migration. The skin of the foot can now be prepared and the colloid injected. The patient should not ambulate until the block is worn off.

III. Scalp

Shave the area to be injected. Use surgical scissors to cut the hair before shaving. Tape can be used to keep the other hair in close proximity to the site away from the intended injection site. The skin of the scalp is difficult to inject therefore the needle tends to penetrate slightly deeper but should be kept in the intradermal site. Contamination of the injection is a real problem; hence assuring good coverage by a sheet around the injection site is required. Care must be given to avoid any leakage from the injection since it can be a source of significant contamination.

IV. Ear

The pinna of the ear heals very well from an excisional biopsy and the actual resection site may be difficult to find. We ask the surgeon to define the exact site of the biopsy. The injection is carried out at two sites: one above and one below the biopsy site. The skin is quite loose, thus the amount of anesthesia and colloid are generally increased in volume. Great care needs to be taken to prevent a blowout of the injection. Preventing contamination of the site is of utmost importance.

V. Trunk

Midline melanomas can be problematic because the tracer can go to almost any basin: axillary, groin or even the supraclavicular region. We have had a patient where the radiocolloid entered the abdominal nodes. Uren has previously described an analogous experience. Intransit nodes can also be found. Uren [1996] pointed out the area of drainage to the triangular intermuscular space and that attention needed to be given to this region. Imaging from the posterior projection would be important in this area of potential involvement.

Areas of Caution:
1. Avoid injecting into very indurated areas. There may be no passage of tracer to the SLN.
2. Avoid injecting in areas of infection. Discuss the situation with the surgeon. The procedure and surgery may be delayed or cancelled.
3. Avoid contamination. Contamination of the skin can be quite confusing by the patterns of lines and spots that can mimic lymphatic channels and lymph nodes.
4. Before injecting near the eye, place a patch of gauze over the eye.
5. Make sure that the correct area is being injected. Review the chart, and if not sure call the surgeon. Sometimes data is lacking on the request.
6. Beware of the contaminated gauze. A small amount of residual tracer on the gauze can create havoc in imaging the nodes. We have the found the most frequent cause of contamination is the gauze used to cover the injection site.
7. With an intradermal injection, movement of radiotracer should be observed in 10 minutes. Reinjection of the site should be considered after this period of time. Particularly in injections of the extremities, lymphatic channels and SLNs have been seen almost immediately after the patient has been injected.

BREAST CANCER

There are a variety of ways to perform lymphoscintigraphy for breast cancer. Different techniques will be discussed below.

Parenchymal Injections – Palpable Masses

Prior to injection, place a warm moist towel over the breast containing the mass. Inject at four quadrants around the palpable mass. Miner [1998] used ultrasound guidance to assist in localizing the needle for injection. Prepare skin as usual and give local anesthesia to skin as described above. Generally, a 1.5-inch 21-gauge needle is sufficient to give the injection into the breast. The needle tip lying next to the tumor or biopsy site can be palpated through the skin. If injection is given into the biopsy site or tumor, there will be a great deal of resistance. Back off a bit, repalpate, then inject. The patient will experience a dull ache, that will fade within about ten minutes. At four sites around the tumor or resection site give one to two ccs of radiocolloid per site using at total dose of 500 to 1000 uCis of filtered Tc99m sulfur colloid. Larger breasts receive more volume. After the injection is done, be careful to avoid, tracer leaking out of the injection site. Apply pressure to the area as needed. Contamination of the area can occur by the leakage from the injection site (Figure 3). Cover the area with gauze. Have the patient massage the breast with her contralateral gloved hand for about 3 to 4 minutes. Begin imaging. The time required for the radiotracer to enter the sentinel node varies. Channels to these node(s) are not always seen but can be prominent (Figure 4a and Figure 4b). If the patient is going to surgery the same day, at least 3 hours should be allotted to visualize the sentinel node. Anecdotal evidence suggests that patients with smaller breasts have more rapid appearance of the sentinel node, and lymphatic channels are more frequently seen. The success rate of locating the sentinel node varies, but is in the range of 80 to 90% [Krag 1998, Hill 1999, Linehan 1999a]. In some of our patients, the node may not be seen until the next day.

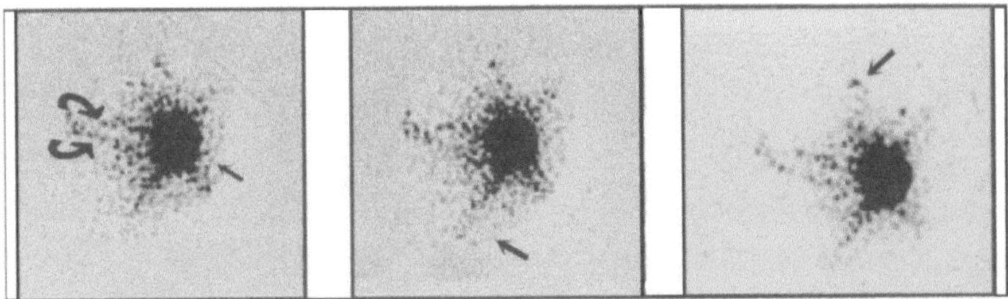

Figure 3. These three panels are from an injection into the right breast. The left panel shows two rounded arrows (A) pointing to what appears to be two separate channels. These findings represent contamination from the parenchymal injection. The radiocolloid has leaked from the injection site causing the problem. The middle panel shows the two channels and the injection site (dark area) and septal flare. Septal flare is the result of penetration of the septa of the collimator by gamma rays and gives the linear lines noted (D). The right panel shows the sentinel node(C).

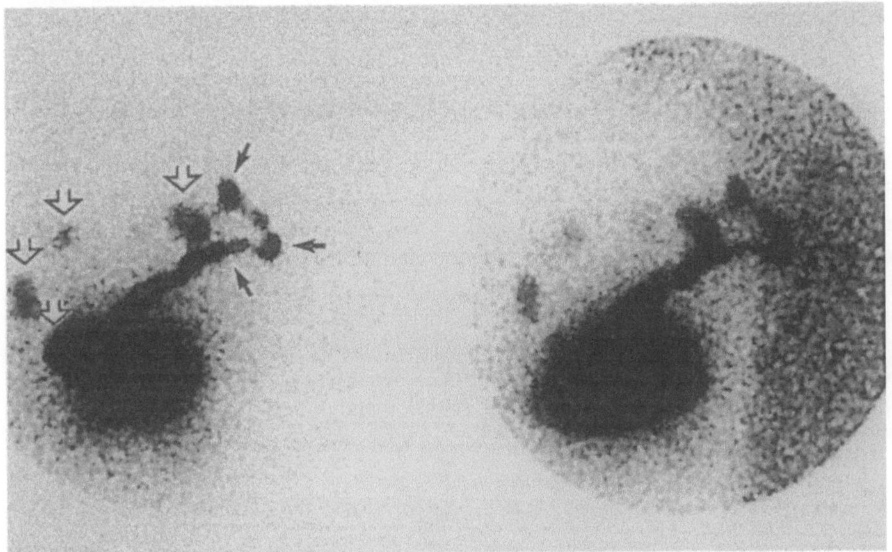

Figure 4a. The image on the left is from a parenchymal injection into the left breast. Very prominent channels are noted (dark closed arrows). Where the channels change direction, there is prominent bulbous activity related to seeing activity end on. The nodes in the axilla and internal mammary areas are show with open arrows. The images are quite dark resulting in a photographic ballooning pattern. The image on the right is the transmission study.

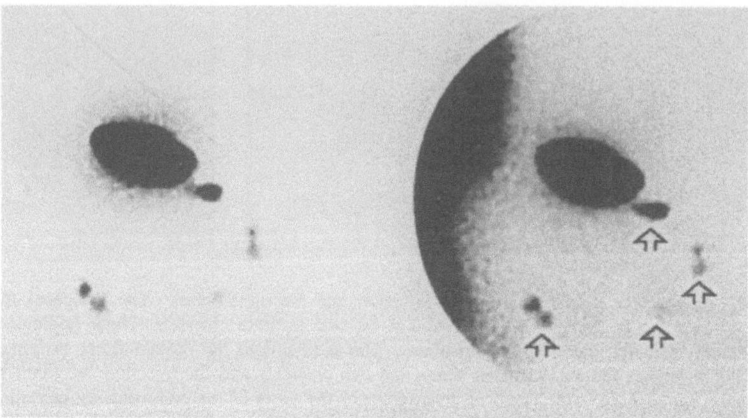

Figure 4b. One hour later, after the channels have had an opportunity to clear, the axillary and internal mammary nodes are easily seen (open arrows).

Doting [2000] used intralesional injections resulting in significant reduction of ballooning effects associated with a large volume of radioactivity.

Parenchymal Injections - Nonpalpable Areas (Mammographic findings)
The injection of the above colloid needs to be done in conjunction with mammography. The radiologists should be asked to place needles straddling the mammographic abnormality. Generally, spinal needles are used in the process. Two needles are required to inject four quadrants. The radiologist should also be asked to place the needles at the end of the calcification on either side of the area in question. The needles should be placed side to side rather than up and down. Needles in a side by side position are much safer as the patients are transported to Nuclear Medicine. At the advice of the radiologists, pull the needles back to inject the other quadrants. Remove the needles after injecting.

Skin Injections
Veronesi, Linehan, Borgstein and Klimberg [Veronesi 1997, Linehan 1999a, Linehan 1999b, Borgstein 1997, Borgstein 1998, Klimberg 1999] use alternative injection techniques to locate the axillary sentinel node. Specifically, Veronesi and Lineham use subdermal (subcutaneous) or intradermal injections, respectively. Klimberg [1999] used a periareolar injection blue dye to locate the sentinel node and found excellent correlation with a simultaneous injection of radiocolloid in the breast. Borgstein [1997, 2000] used parenchymal injection of radiocolloid with periareolar injection of blue dye and found excellent correlation with axillary SLN. Borgstein [2000] found 15 % of their patients had internal mammary nodes and in only 3 of 220 patient was the SLN only in the internal mammary chain. At Sloan Kettering Memorial Cancer Center, Linehan developed a protocol in which patients were injected around the tumor with blue dye and in the skin with unfiltered Tc99m sulfur colloid above the tumor. The Sloan Kettering investigators found that in the vast majority of patients, the sentinel node was found by both techniques to be the same node. Grant [1959] found a rich circumareolar plexus that drains the deeper

lymphatics of the breast. Observation of the skin injections and localization in SLNs confirm Grant's findings. Skin injections do not show the internal mammary chain. Data from Vendrell-Torne [1972] showed that periareolar injections could go to the internal mammary chain. However, a more recent work with periareolar injection of colloid and blue dye has not shown activity in the internal mammary chain [Klimberg 1999, Kern 200]. Concurrently, in our experience with melanomas of the chest wall, we have never seen internal mammary nodes and the published works by those performing skin injection in breast cancer patients have not noted internal mammary nodes. Our findings are in agreement with the published works by the investigators performing skin injections in breast cancer patients. If the internal mammary nodes are to be evaluated, a peritumoral injection is necessary.

Our group has chosen to use intradermal injections as suggested by Linehan. Correlations in about a dozen patients with parenchymal and intradermal injection of radiocolloid have shown the same sentinel node(s). These findings are similar to those found by Roumen [1999].

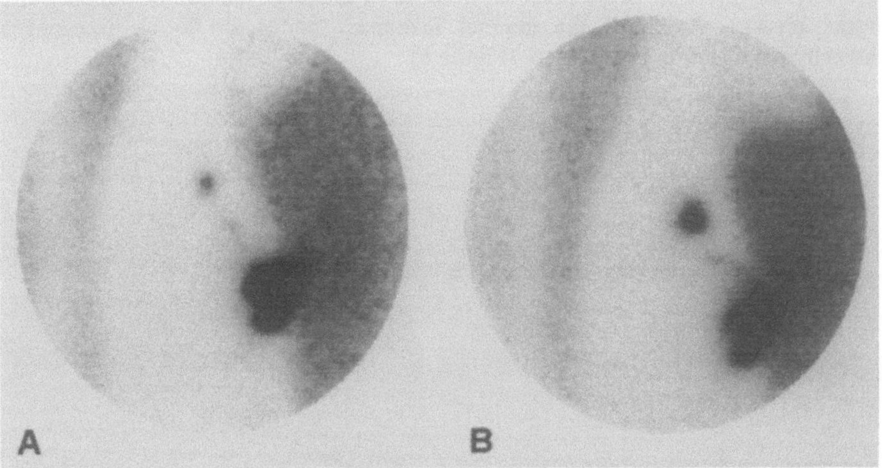

Figure 5. The left panel is from an injection into the right breast and the right axillary sentinel node. A faint channel can be seen. The right panel is from the skin injection done immediately after imaging the parenchymal injection. The sentinel node is the same node. This finding was confirmed on other views. From: Morita ET, et al. Principles and controversies in lymphoscintigraphy with emphasis on breast cancer. In: Leong SPL, Wong JH, editors. Surgical Clinics of North America: Sentinel Lymph Nodes in Human Solid Cancer. Philadelphia: W.B. Saunders, 2000; 80(6), with permission.

The intradermal injection of filtered radiocolloid is the same as in melanoma patients. With the patient in the supine projection, a single injection is given over the palpable area or mammographic calcification (marks made by radiologists). Imaging is begun immediately after the injection.

First, the intradermal injections have a much higher count rate in the sentinel node as compared to a parenchymal injection. The sentinel node is usually seen within 10 minutes and often immediately after the injection. Secondly, the problem of the "shine through effect" is reduced. The "shine through effect" is a result of the injection site ballooning its activity into the axilla. A third advantage is that the patient can be studied in the afternoon and go to surgery the next morning since the amount of radioactivity in the sentinel node is greater by a skin injection when compared with a intraparenchymal injection. Despite decay of the Tc99m colloid, sufficient radioacitivy remains to find the SLN(s) intraoperatively. Generally, there is a higher degree of success via an intradermal injection as compared to a parenchymal injection. With a parenchymal injection a delayed 24-hour study might not show a SLN. This would delay surgery. A fourth advantage is the use of a small piece of 1/8-inch thick lead on top of the gauze covering the injection site. This reduces the septal penetration of the collimator. The lead does not impede the passage of radiocolloid to the sentinel node. Using lead for a parenchymal injection is not practical because of the large amount of radioactivity in the breast. Again, if the internal mammary nodes are to be assessed a parenchymal injection is necessary (Figure 6).

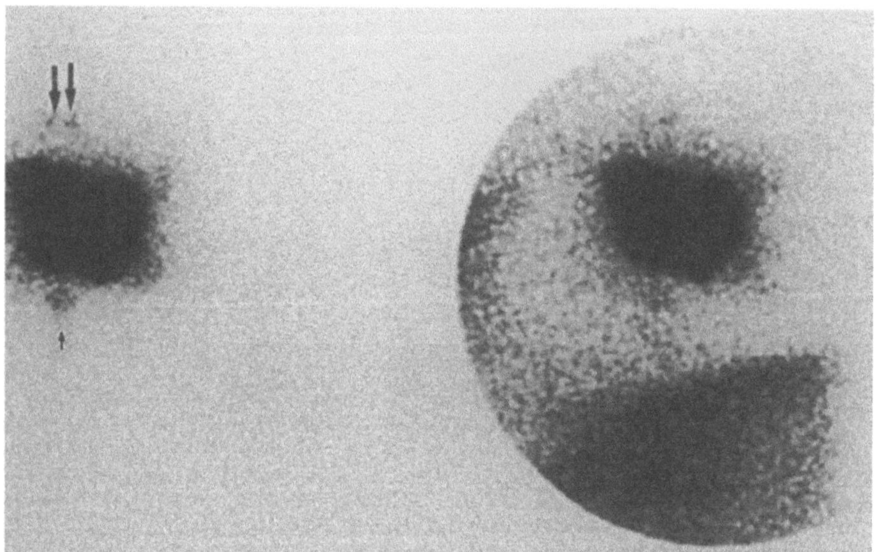

Figure 6. A parenchymal injection of radiocolloid in the right breast shows both lower sentinel axillary node (smaller dark arrow) and two internal mammary sentinel nodes (large dark arrows). The panel on the right is the transmission study.

DETECTION OF THE SENTINEL NODE

There are two major pieces of equipment used for lymphoscintigraphy, the gamma camera and the gamma probe.

Gamma Camera [Anger 1967, Simmons 1996, Gunter 1996]

This device is able to image the radioactivity injected into a patient. Because the radioactivity is not confounded by background activity in the surrounding tissues, lymphatic channels and nodes are easily seen. The gamma camera is equipped with electronic device, a pulse height analyzer, which are able to tell the primary photon of Tc99m from scattered irradiation. When a gamma photon passes through tissue it may interact and cause scattered photons. These scattered photons do not come from the injection site but reflect the position of the interaction with tissue and may have come from several inches from the injection site. In the process of scatter, the primary energy of Tc99m is degraded and possesses less energy. The pulse height analyzer separates the true activity coming from a patient's injection site, channels and SLN and eliminates those photons that are from scattered sources.

A device called a collimator is placed in front of the gamma camera's crystal to give precise localization of radioactivity emanating from the patient. Unlike light radiation, gamma photons cannot be bent and focused. The purpose of the collimator is to permit only gamma photons coming perpendicularly to the detector to be recorded. The collimator is made of lead with multiple holes that are perpendicular to the gamma camera crystal. The lead eliminates almost all gamma photons not perpendicular to the gamma camera's crystal. A phenomenon called "septal penetration" causes a flare defect on the images due to gamma photons penetrating the leaded septa of the collimator. The problem with flare is that it can obscure the images of the node. A collimator with more lead can eliminate this problem. An alternative is to use a pinhole collimator. The pinhole will eliminate all flare. The pinhole collimator is a cone shaped device that is place on the gamma camera's detector. In concept it is analogous to a pinhole camera. There is a single hole in the collimator. The pinhole can be placed a few inches from the area to be studied. This collimator is useful when the injection site is very close to the basin in question, such as an upper outer quadrant of the breast. With the use of the normal collimator, there can be a pronounced shine effect as well as septal flare that make imaging the questioned basin difficult to evaluate. The pinhole collimator eliminates these confounding effects.

An integral part of the gamma camera is the persistence oscilloscope (P-scope). This device permits the Nuclear Medicine physician the opportunity to see the images in real time. Generally, it lacks good detail but is helpful in marking the SLN. These marks help the surgeon to locate the sentinel node with the gamma probe (see below). Some P-scopes are very user friendly and others are not. The greater ease in use of the P-scope allows marks to be placed quite easily on the patient. It should be noted that some investigators do not use imaging in locating the sentinel node [Krag 1999]. The surgeons in our institution find the localization helpful and feel that the time in surgery is reduced.

Gamma Probe

The gamma probe [Britten 1997, Hoffman 1999, Schneebaum 1999, Zanzonico 2000] is a hand held device that permits the surgeon to locate the SLN in the operating room. The detector of the gamma probe is made of materials, such as sodium iodide or cadmium-zinc-telluride that interacts with the gamma photon from the patient and records this interaction as a count. The detector is designed to count the activity that is directly in front of it. There is sufficient lateral shielding to eliminate photons coming from the side. The concept of the inverse square law is important in localizing the SLN (Figure 7). As the detector is moved closer to the area of

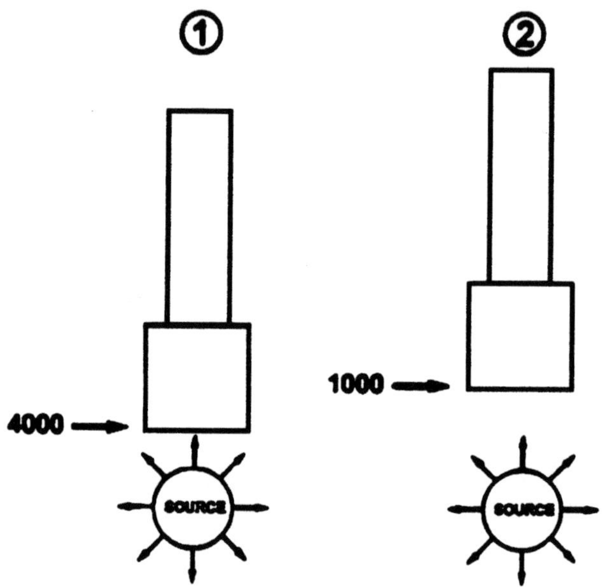

Figure 7. Inverse square law. With radioactive source at position "1", the gamma probe counts in this example are 4000 counts. By moving the probe to twice the distance form the source, to position "2", the counts decrease to 1000 counts. The importance of the inverse square law is utilizing the concept when using the gamma probe in a clinical setting. In probing for the SLN, by moving the gamma closer or farther will give dramatic changes in the counts. The law applies in radiation safety by decreasing counts by a factor of four with a doubling the distance away from the source. From: Morita ET, et al. Principles and controversies in lymphoscintigraphy with emphasis on breast cancer. In: Leong SPL, Wong JH, editors. Surgical Clinics of North America: Sentinel Lymph Nodes in Human Solid Cancer. Philadelphia: W.B. Saunders, 2000;80(6), with permission.

radioactivity, the counts will increase as a function of the distance. For example, the counts at 2 inches from the SLN may be at 1000 counts/second but when moved to 1 inch, the counts will increase to 4000 counts/second. Moving the detector twice the distance closer increases the counts by a factor of four not two. Radiation is given off as a sphere of activity. The closer the detector is to the source of radiation, the larger the angle is which the detector subtends. On occasions, the gamma probe may require a collimator placed over the front of the detector. This narrows the field of view of the probe and can be quite helpful when one is trying to separate two nodes that are close together (Figure 8). Furthermore, the collimator on the probe is useful when the injection site and SLN are in close proximity. Gamma probes have discriminators, which separate the primary gamma photons from scattered, degraded photons. The gamma probes systems are equipped with both audible signals as well as eleectronic count displays. Both are useful in the operating room.

Separating and counting the nodes on a tabletop after removal from the patient is useful since additional nodes may be found. Statistical evaluation of the data is useful in determining which node is the hottest. To accomplish this task, each node is counted for 3-4 seconds. The total counts of nodes are determined by multiplying the count rate (counts/second) by the time counted (seconds). For example, a counted node has a count rate of 2500 counts/second and is counted for 4 seconds. The total count is 10,000 counts. The standard deviation of the count is calculated by taking the square root of the count. In this example, the standard deviation is

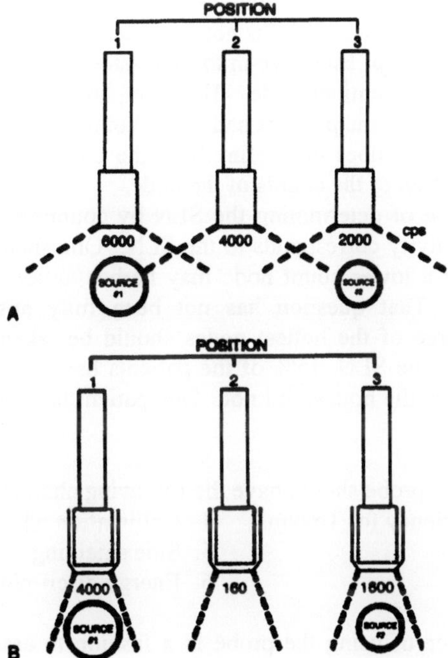

Figure 8. The gamma probe with and without a collimator are seen in A and B. Without the collimator (A) sources cannot be separated because moving from position "1" through "3" the counts are such as not to be able to define the sources as being separate. With the collimator in place (B), the two sources can be easily separated because of the counts differences are distinct. The collimator limits the angle the gamma detector thus reducing the counts as well as allowing the detector to separate the two sources. From: Morita ET, et al. Principles and controversies in lymphoscintigraphy with emphasis on breast cancer. In: Leong SPL, Wong JH, editors. Surgical Clinics of North America: Sentinel Lymph Nodes in Human Solid Cancer. Philadelphia: W.B. Saunders, 2000; 80(6), with permission.

100, the square root of 10,000. Adding or subtracting two standard deviations (200 counts) from the total count represents a 95% confidence level that a repeated counting will result in a count between 9800 to 10,200. Three standard deviations (+/-300 counts) represent a 99% confidence level that a repeated count would be from 9700 to 10,300. Another node in this area with a count of 2000 counted for 4 seconds (total count = 8000 counts) could be separated statistically to determine whether the two nodes are significantly different from each other. In this example, there is a statistical difference that the count of 10,000 is hotter than the node with the count of 8000. Where there is overlap of standard deviations, the two counts may not be clearly defined as to one being hotter than the other may. The standard deviation of the counts can be used to determine if there is a statistical difference. Counting the nodes for only one second would decrease the differentiation among nodes. For this reason, counting for four seconds is recommended to ensure that nodes can be differentiated from each other. If a node has a lower count, counting for a longer period of time is required to adequately define the different nodes statistically. Counting nodes in this fashion provides precision in the separation of two nodes.

By counting nodes in this fashion, we have found that fifteen percent of the time, the node bearing the tumor (SLN) is not the hottest. Porter [2000] and Morton [1999b] recommend the use of Blue Dye in the assessment with lymphoscintigraphy to determine which is the sentinel node. However, in his study with Blue Dye, Porter found that only 1% of the patients had a less hot node containing tumor when the hottest did not. Porter does not define how the counts were determined and gives no standard deviation of the counts of the node.

The importance of determining the SLN by counting nodes ex-vivo is to determine how radioactivity corresponds to the SLN. One should not remove only the hottest node, since a lower count node may harbor tumor. How many nodes should be removed? That question has not been fully answered but in our experience, at least three of the hottest nodes should be taken. In our series of patients with tumors in the SLN, 15% of the patients had nodes with less activity had tumor present where the hottest did not. One patient had the third hottest node harboring tumor.

In summary, the gamma probe should have the following characteristics:

1. Good counting efficiency for Tc99m
2. Small diameter
3. lateral shielding
4. Collimation when needed
5. Side shielding
6. Energy discrimination

The importance of using the probe in a fashion to assure that the counts obtained are statistical significant and how these counts relate to the sentinel nodes.

IMAGING PROTOCOL

General Comments on Imaging

When observing with the P-Scope, lymphatic channels should be seen within minutes after the injection. Most P-Scopes permit acquisition of data for better detail. As previously mentioned, some P-scopes are more "user friendly" than others are. As details are observed, channels will be visualized as the radiotracer leaves the injection site. The nodal basin in question is usually seen within ten minutes. If nodal basins and channels are not seen, one should consider reinjection of the site. If the injection is in a limb, exercising the limb may help move the tracer from the injection site.

In older patients with very thin, parchment-like skin, forming a good wheal for injection can be very difficult. A slightly larger wheal may be necessary.

MELANOMA

After injection of the radiocolloid described above, the following protocol is suggested.

Lower extremity

Place the camera in the area of the expected basin. Set the computer to acquire images in a dynamic fashion to observe the channels entering the lymph node basin. Generally, the system can be set for 10 minutes. Use a matrix of 64 x 64 or 128 x 128, depending on your system. The acquisition parameters are likewise dependent on the system available. Acquiring data at 15-second intervals for ten minutes will permit dynamic evaluation when played back in a dynamic fashion. Depending on the activity found in the channels, summing of these intervals could be combined to increase the quality and detail of the dynamic images. This summing process can provide a higher degree of confidence in determining the channel's relationship to the radioactive nodes. The channels are important because they define the SLN. At times, the channels may end in different nodes resulting in finding separate, multiple SLNs. Image all the areas from the injection site to the primary basin of involvement since intransit node can be missed if the path of radiocolliod is not followed.

In areas below the knee, evaluation of the popliteal area is important since nodes at this site can occur about 10% of the time. The bolus of radioactivity in the lymphatic channels can be followed and if necessary, the position of the detector can be moved to better evaluate a basin. Channels may be in series or parallel.

Static images are obtained after the dynamic set. A transmission study is done after the dynamic study to obtain a body outline of the nodal basin (Figure 9). Images are collected on the computer in matrix of 128 x 128 or 256 x 256. Generally, images are collected from 2 to 4 minutes depending on the amount of activity in the node(s). In the groin and popliteal areas, in addition to the anterior view, lateral images are also obtained. The lateral view gives some indication whether some of the nodes may lay deeper in the iliac chain. After the images are collected, the nodes found are marked in the anterior projection. Marking is done by using an external Tc99m point source and moving the source until the radioactive lymph node is directly over the radioactive marking source. The skin is marked with gentian violet over the node. This is accomplished by using the P-scope previously described.

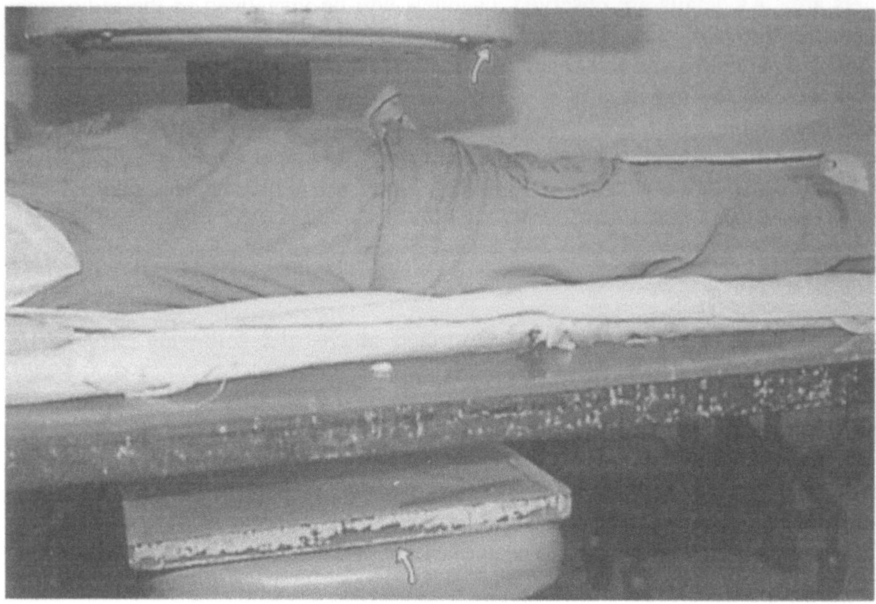

Figure 9. The use of a sheet source of Tc 99m in a saline reservoir or a sealed source of Cobalt 57 can provide an anatomic outline of the body. The source is under the patient and the detector above the patient. About 5 mCis in the saline source is sufficient to give well defined body contours in 30 seconds (see Figure 2c).

Upper extremity melanomas

The technique of imaging the upper extremity is similar to that of the lower extremity. The methods of recording data are also similar. For sites below the elbow, imaging is similar to those of the lower extremity. The epitrochlear nodes are difficult to isolate with the gamma camera so we place a gentian violet skin mark at the general level for the surgeon to locate the node in the operating room by going circumferentially around the marked site. The axillary nodes are defined in anterior, lateral and 45-degree projections with appropriate marks. The greater the separation of these marks, the deeper the node. These multiple views meet at a point, which locate the SLN.

Trunk melanomas

Melanomas in the trunk can travel to almost any basin. Start imaging the injection site and move the detector to follow the activity as its channels declare the location. On occasions, a melanoma located laterally may be best imaged from the lateral or oblique positions. Generally with trunk melanomas, image all potential basins (Figure 10, 11, 12a, 12b).

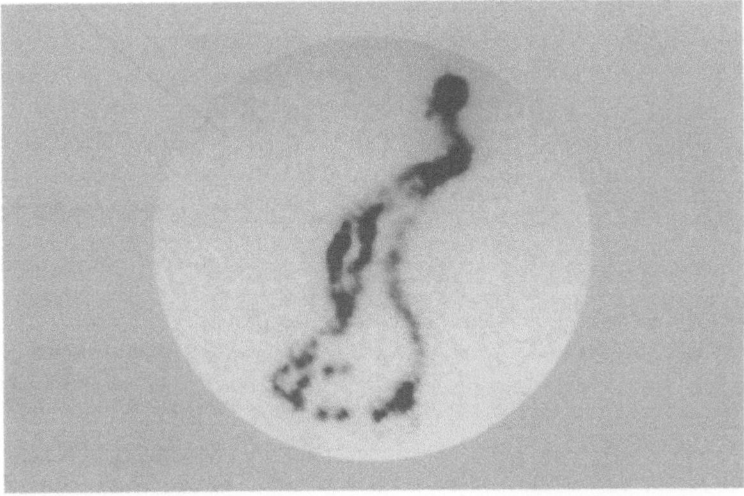

Figure 10. Arrow "C" shows the injection site in a patient with a melanoma of the abdominal wall. The rectangular area represents a piece of lead over the injection site. From the injection site, there are two distinct channels (parallel) moving cephalad toward the left axilla. Arrow "B "shows three channels (open arrows). Moving toward the axilla, the channels coalesce into what appears to be one channel (Arrow "A") as it enters the axilla. Observations with Blue dye showed this channel to be a single channel. Lymphoscintigraphy is limited in its resolution as to be unable to clearly define the channels as a single channel or three closely related channels moving side by side.

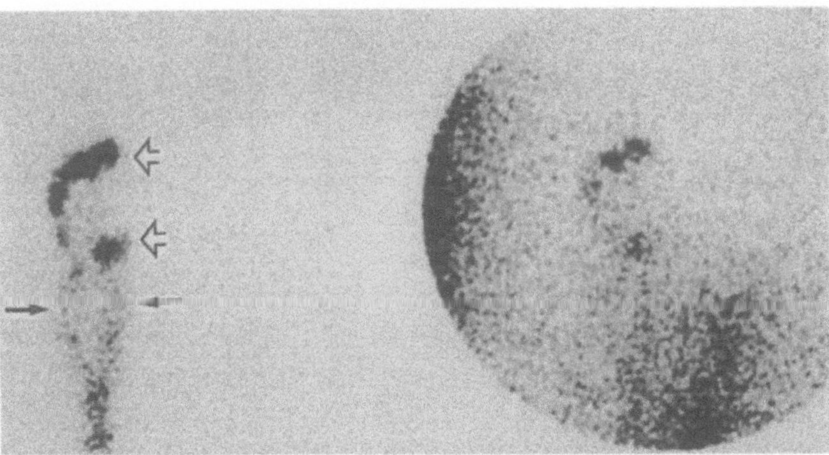

Figure 11. The images on the left show two separate channels (closed arrows) and two separate sentinel lymph nodes (open arrows) in the right groin. Without seeing the channels entering the nodes, the first more proximal node to the injection site might have mistakenly considered the only sentinel node. Lymphoscintigraphy in this patient defined that there were two separate sentinel nodes. By only the using the gamma probe, the distinction could not have been made. The panel on the right shows the transmission study.

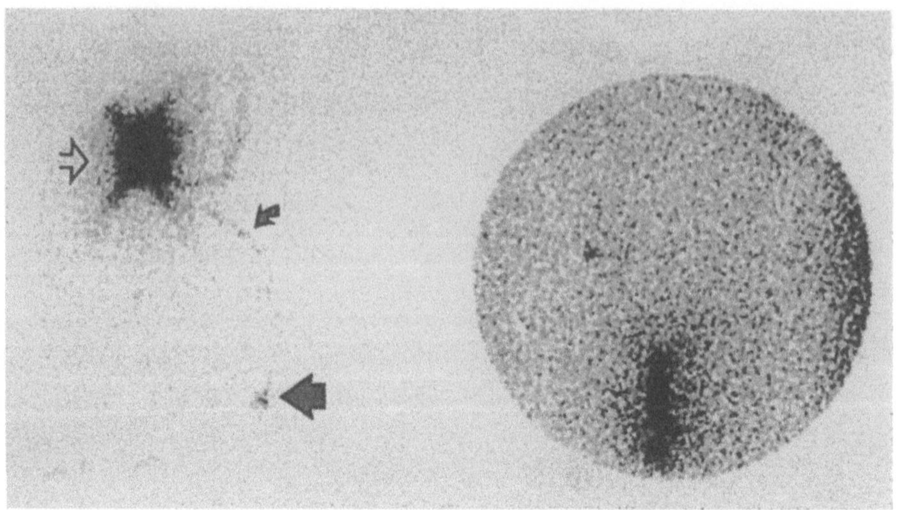

Figure 12a. The injection site (open arrow) was made in the right flank. Three distinct channels (dark arrows) can be seen moving cephalad toward the right axilla. They appear to merge into one channel as it enters the right axilla to the sentinel node. The curved darkened arrow shows an additional channel extending caudally. The transmission studies show the position of the injection site and channels with respect to the body outline.

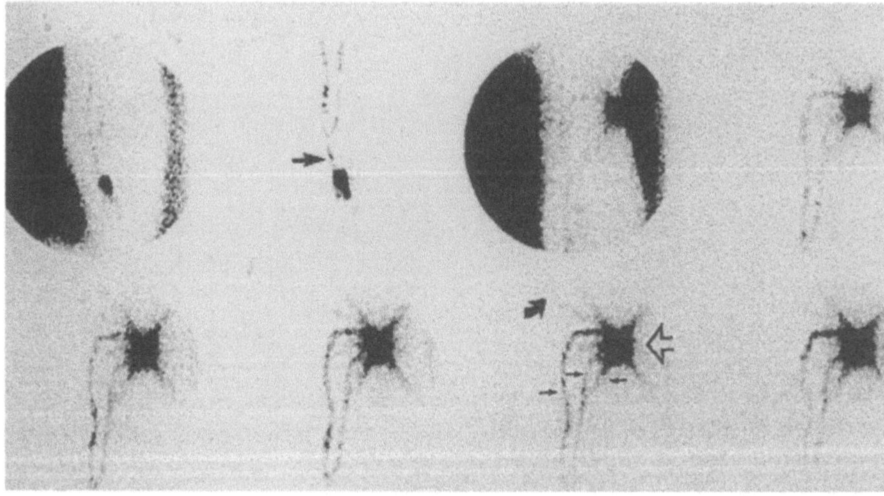

Figure 12b.   The injection site in the right flank is shown as an open arrow. The curved darkened arrow show the single channel moving toward the right groin. The large dark arrow points to the sentinel node in the right groin. The panel on the right is the transmission study.

Head, neck and scalp melanomas (Figure 13)

The head, neck and scalp are the most difficult to evaluate. The injection site and basin may be quite close to each other. The use of the pinhole collimator under this circumstance can be quite helpful. In this area, marks are usually made in the lateral projection. For scalp areas, anterior or posterior views are helpful for localization (Figure 14a and Figure 14b). In the area of the pinna of the ear, moving the ear can be helpful in determining whether the node is anterior or posterior to the ear. Moving the pinna of the ear can reveal a node posteriorly placed, near the mastoid that has been obscured by the injection site.

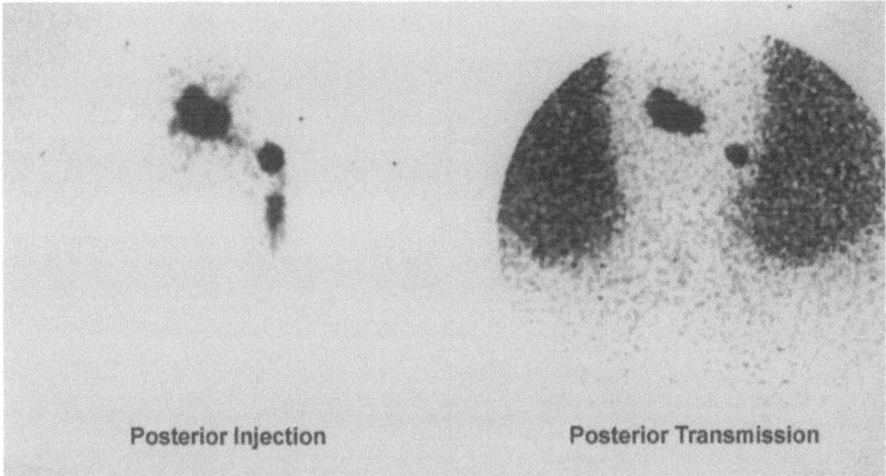

Figure 13. The image on the left shows the left -midline posterior scalp injection site and a channel moving down into the right posterior cervical chain. There is a pass through node below the first node. The transmission study is shown on the left.

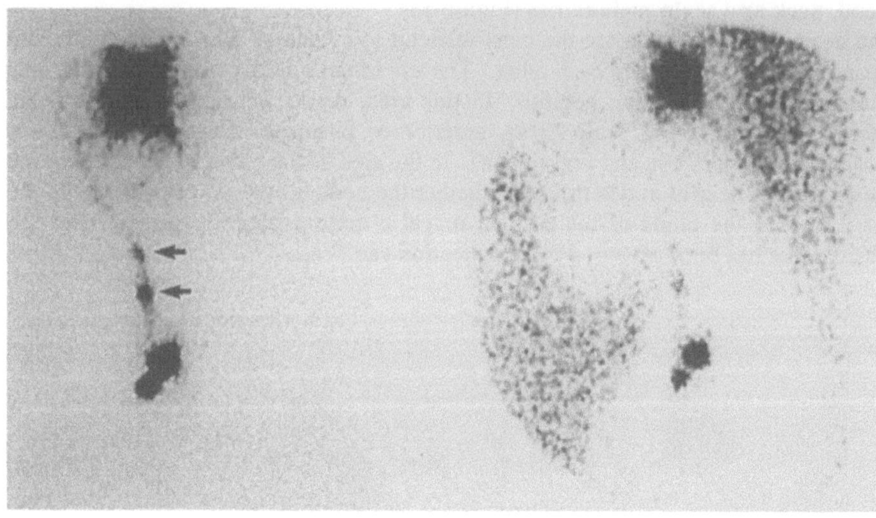

Figure 14a. The left image shows the left lateral projection of a posterior scalp melanoma injection site with several channels coalescing into one (arrows). The arrows show two distinct focal areas as the channel extends into the left axilla. The focal areas noted prior to the axillary sentinel nodes, could be mistaken for lymph nodes.

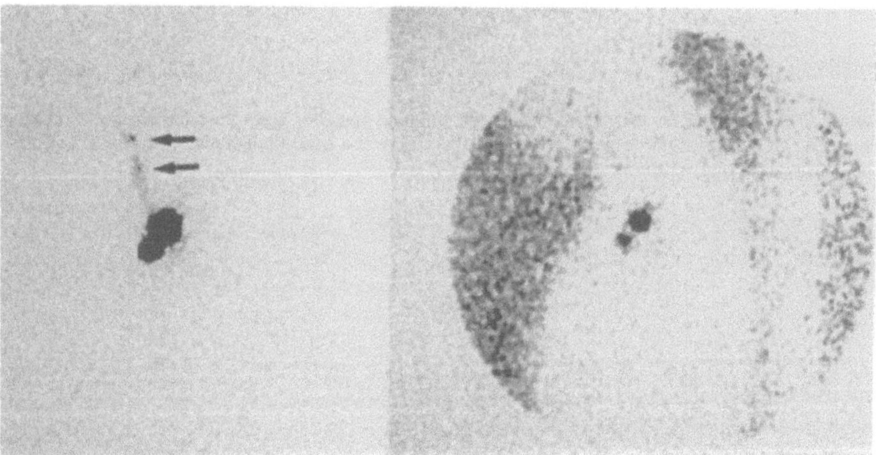

Figure 14b. This image is a continuation of Figure 14a. On delayed images done an hour later shows significant clearing of the initial intense areas noted in Figure 10a. These areas (arrows) represent bulbous areas in the lymphatic channels that clear over time. These should not be mistaken for intransit nodes.

BREAST CARCINOMA

Parenchymal injection

A dynamic set as described above is suggested. Image in the anterior projection. Channels can be seen but not as consistently as those noted in melanoma patients. When the SLN is close proximity to the injection site, moving the breast away from the SLN can be helpful (Figure 15). The procedure takes about one hour to accomplish with views done in multiple projections of the axilla. If internal mammary nodes are seen, they are marked in the anterior projection. On occasion, delayed films may be required. About three hours should be allotted prior to the scheduled surgery.

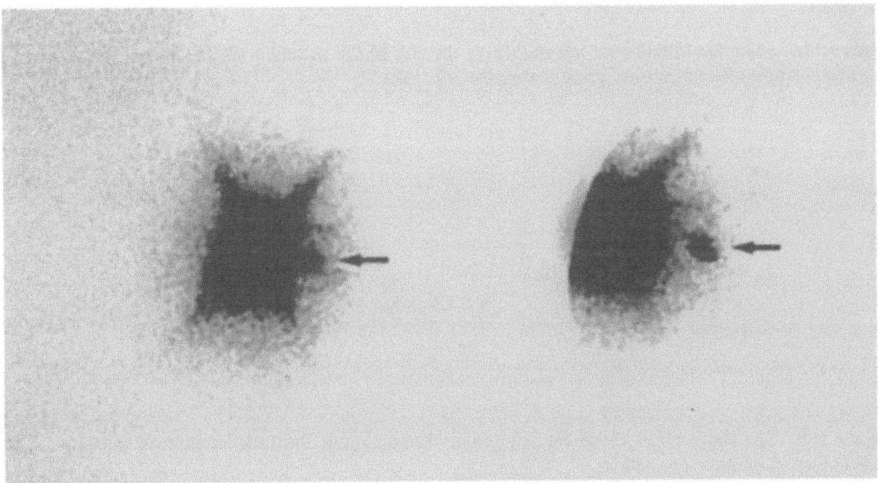

Figure 15. The image on the left is the parenchymal left breast injection with the arrow pointing to the sentinel lymph node in the left axilla. The image on the right was taken after the patient moved her breast medially. This image shows the sentinel lymph node (arrow) with greater separation and definition.

When the injection is close to the axillary basin, the breast can be displaced to better visualize the sentinel node. Pinhole images can be quite helpful when the injection site is very close to the axillary basin. Marking can be difficult however because the area to be imaged is small. A general area can be marked as to the location of SLN and the surgeon advised.

Intradermal injection

A dynamic set is obtained as described. The injection of the tracer is placed above the tumor mass or mammographic finding. The gauze-covered injection site can be covered with a small piece of lead. This reduces the activity in the imaged area and reduces the "shine effect" of the injection site. The lead does not impede the passage of tracer through the lymphatic channels. The lead piece is particularly useful in upper-outer quadrant lesions. Since the injection is similar to those of a melanoma study, channels are consistently seen (Figure 16a and Figure 16b).

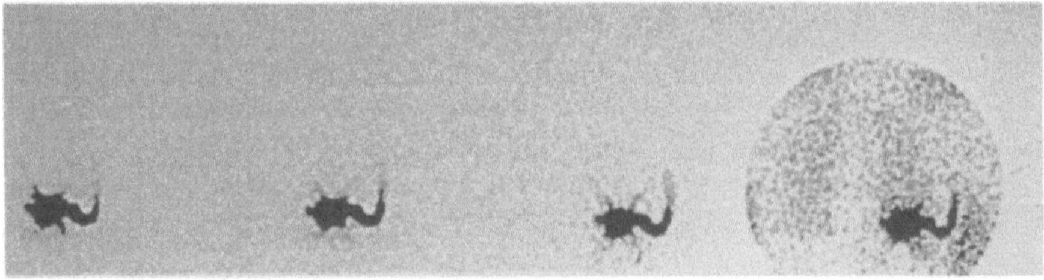

Figure 16a. After the intradermal injection over the site of the patient's left breast primary cancer, a prominent single channel is seen going toward the left axilla.

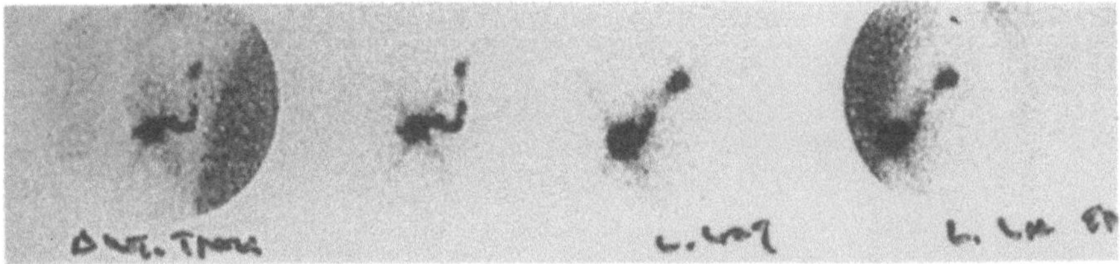

Figure 16b. The above panel shows the left axillary sentinel node from the intradermal injection. The node is seen in multiple projections.

COMPUTER PROCESSING

Dynamic set
The dynamic collection can be summed as a single image to provide more detail of the channels. Review the set for motion artifacts since adding images that are not in the same position on the screen will result in degraded images. Add only those in which motion is not seen. A higher level of confidence can be attained for the channels in relationships to the nodes.

Static images
Images should be of sufficient counts and have a fairly homogeneous texture. The aim should be to have good detail in all the nodes imaged.

Masking
All computer systems permit exclusion of an area by a processing called masking. Usually this is done with a light pen. The area to be excluded from the image is circled and eliminated. Depending on the computer system, the various gradations of counts in the nodes can be seen from the lowest to the highest. When the hottest nodes becomes so dominant as to reduce the visualization of other nodes in the basin, masking of this area will enhance the nodes with lesser activity. Current computer systems have log display scales that permit visualizing a larger count spread (Figure 17). The log scale permits reducing the higher count displays to "fit"

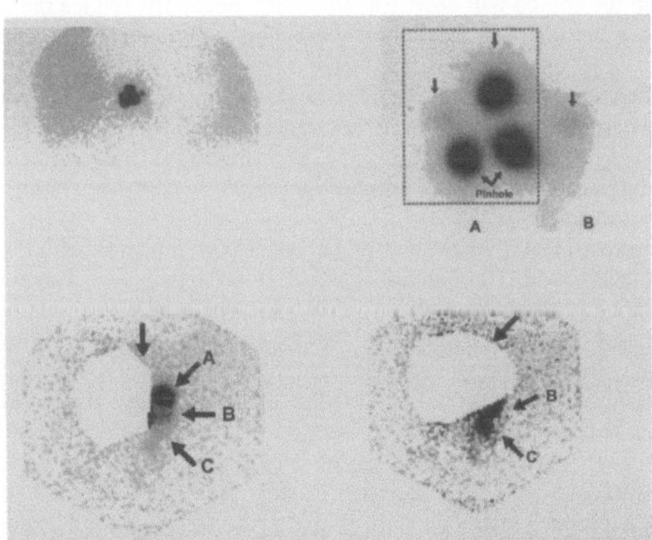

Figure 17. The upper left image shows the injection site in the right lateral projection of a patient with a melanoma of the right upper neck. The panel on the top right is a pinhole image (in the dotted rectangular box, "A") of the injection site. Arrows point to the four injection sites. One injection site is quite faint. Sentinel lymph nodes are seen at "B". The bottom left p nel shows the nodes after of the injection site. with further masking additional nodes are noted in much better detail.

allowing visualization of all the nodes in question. Older systems may not have this function; hence masking becomes more important. With images that are well displayed, a higher level of confidence can be reached when describing a finding. A level of confidence in interpretation of the images can assist the surgeon with the anatomy of the nodes in a given basin.

RADIATION SAFETY

The most important aspect of radiation safety with for lymphoscintigraphy is education. The doses used are extraordinarily small. Advise all members of the team from Nuclear Medicine to Pathology. The patient should be well informed of the procedure, the radiation involved, and what will be accomplished by lymphoscintigraphy. Having in-services education on each section is very important. Answer all questions. Discuss safety protocols and provide a phone number to call if there are questions. The State of California does not require an amendment to the radiologic license to perform lymphoscintigraphy [Department of Health Services 1999].

Three maneuvers can reduce radiation to those involved in the procedure. Two of these are quite practical the third is much less so. The first is understanding the concept of the inverse square law described previously. Radiation is emitted as a sphere of activity. The closer that one is to the source, the larger the angle of the sphere covered. When the distance is doubled, the radiation is reduced not by a factor of two, but by a factor of four, it's the square of the distance. Increasing the distance from the source will decrease radiation. Secondly, reduce the contact time to reduce exposure. This is a common sense approach one use to reduce exposure. A third item is to use shielding to reduce exposure in the operating room suite. From our measurement of the standard doses given, shielding is not necessary. Moving lead shield into a crowded operating room may prove to be a greater physical hazard. From our monitoring the operating room from an injected 400 uCi dose of Tc99m sulfur colloid has been at the periphery of the operating room to be near background levels.

Veronesi [1999] found that at 18 hours post injection of 135 to 270 uCi the dose to the hands in 100 operations to be 450 mrem per year. This is a relatively small exposure to the hands. Barral [1991] showed that when holding a syringe with 20 mCis of Tc99m, the finger in contact with the syringe received a dose of 22,000 mR/hr. In the clinical context of lymphoscintigraphy, the usual dose of 500 uCi would result in a dose rate of 550 mR/hr. In breast tissue, the radiation dose to the surgeon's hand would be reduced because of the absorption of radiation from the injection site by the soft tissues of the breast. From personal discussion with one of our surgeons, SPL, the exposure of this type is at most 30 seconds in a patient with a parenchymal injection of 500 uCi. A 30-second exposure would result in only 0.152 mR. The tumor would be removed with the use of surgical instruments over a period of approximately 40 minutes. At 6 cm from the radioactive injection site resulting a radiation to the hands of only an additional dose of .86 mR. This data is again from the hand dose radiation measured by Barral [1991]. The total dose to the surgeon's hand would be 2.16 mR for the removal of the radioactive breast mass. Studies by Veronesi [1999] and Barral [1991] show the doses to the surgeon's hand to be extraordinarily low. The removal of excisional biopsy or the primary melanoma with 500 uCi at the site would also be very low since most of this removal would be done with forceps.

Monitoring the amount of radiation can be accomplished by placing radiation badges around the operating room at various sites and determining the dose rate in a given circumstance. This provides useful baseline data. This should be done in coordination with the radiation safety officer (RSO). The data would give an idea of the amount of radiation involved in a clinical situation.

Those who come in contact with radioactive materials in the operating room should also be badged. One individual should be designated as the point of contact for the RSO. Radiation monitoring badges will be collected and a new one issued every month. Our monitoring of these badges has not found an alarming amount of exposure.

All surgeons performing sentinel node dissections and other procedures using radioactive materials in the operating room should also be badged. The point of contact for the OR staff will be the point of contact for the surgeons as well. Wearing finger dosimeters would not be practical since they cannot be readily sterilized and would be cumbersome during surgery.

HANDLING AND MONITORING THE SPECIMEN [Fitzgibbons 2000]:

Despite low levels of measured radioactivity, the specimens are isolated for 24 hours and marked as both biologic and radiation samples. The samples will be placed in a similarly labeled lead box with sufficient shielding to provide adequate protection from exposure. A 1/8-inch piece of lead will be sufficient to reduce the levels to background. For melanoma patients, the sample does not be sent for frozen section. If necessary, a complete lymphadenctomy is performed after determining the status of the SLN(s). We have monitored the dissection tables in the Department of Pathology and found them to be at background levels.

For patients with breast cancer, frozen or touch preparations may be necessary to assist the surgeon in determining the need for further resection. Again, we have monitored this area and found background levels at the operative site. The surgical samples from a 400 uCi dose on sample was 9.5 mrem/hour on contact with the sample and 2.5 mrem/hour at 6.5 cm. Since the pathologist uses only small amounts of tissue, the radiation dose is substantially less than the amounts mentioned above as measured by the UCSF/MSH RSO. Pathologists and personnel in Pathology at UCSF/MZH have been badged and exposure has been close to background.

PREGNANT WOMEN

Pregnant women who need lymphoscintigraphy should not be absolutely excluded from study. The dose to the fetus from a parenchymal injection into the breast or skin would be quite low [Russell 1997]. The dose of the injection into the breast could be reduced to decrease the exposure to the developing fetus. For example, a parenchymal breast injection of 500 uCi Tc99m sulfur colloid with the assumption that the entire dose entered the liver and spleen, the fetus would receive a dose of 5. mrem [Current radiation 1975]. The fetal radiation in which the dose staying in the breast would be much lower because of the distance from the fetus would be greater. Pregnancy, per se, should not be an absolute contraindication for lymphoscintigraphy [Morita 2000]. A frank discussion of the amount of radiation involved and other risks to the fetus would be of great importance to the pregnant patient.

To review: educate all the personnel involved with the technique and amount of radiation involved. The doses to those in Nuclear Medicine, surgery, and pathology are at very low levels. Contamination has been monitored and has not been a problem in the operating room or pathology. Once baseline work has been done, we monitor as needed or if there are questions from the OR staff.

CONCLUSION

In this chapter we have provided suggestions and techniques that have been accrued from our experience with lymphoscintigraphy. Each hospital and personnel may have different requirements. From a practical standpoint, the above methods have been used for several years. We feel comfortable with our methodology. Full understanding of the inverse square law will lead to more efficient use of the gamma probe and radiation safety. If there is poor communication or lack of support in any part of the process, the program will not be successful. For a program to work well all physicians involved with lymphoscintigraphy should visit the departments of Nuclear Medicine, surgery and Pathology to observe first hand what happens in each department. An important factor is the cooperatioin of all disciplines involved in defining the sentinel lymph node.

The author would like to thank Mr. Ray Darbyshire, CNMT for his technical expertise.

REFERENCES

Anger HO. Radioisotope cameras. In:Hine GJ, editor. Instrumentation in Nuclear Medicine. New York: Academic Press; 1967. p.485-552.

Barrall RC. Radiation safety consideration for meducal use of technetium-99m. In: Kereiakes JG, editor. Biophyscial Aspects: Medical Use of Technetium-99m. American Association of Physicists in Medicine, Topical Review Series, 1991, 108-149.

Borgstein P, Pijpers R, Comans EF, et al. Sentinel lymph node biopsy in breast cancer: guidelines and pitfalls of lymphoscintigraphy and gamma probe detection. Journal American College of Surgeons 1998;186(3):275-283

Borgstein PJ, Meijer S, Pijpers R. Intradermal blue dye to identify sentinel lymph-node in breast cancer. Lancet 1997;349(9066):1668-9

Britten AJ. A method to evaluate intra-operative gamma probes for sentinel lymph node localisation. European Journal of Nuclear Medicine 1999;26(2):76-83

Cabanas RM. An approach for the treatment of penile carcinoma. Cancer 1977;39(2):456-466

Current radiation dose estimate to humans with various liver conditions from technetium 99m colloid, MIRD dose estimate report #3. Journal of Nuclear Medicine 1975;16:108

Daniels GH. Introduction to the thyroid diseases, physical examination of the thyroid gland. In: Braverman LE, Utiger RD, et al., editors. Werner and Ingbar's the thyroid: a fundamental and clinical text. 6th ed. Philadelpia: Lippincott; 1991. p.576.

De Cicco C, Cremonesi M, Chinol M, et al. Optimization of axillary lymphoscintigraphy to detect the sentinel node in breast cancer. Tumori 1997;83(2):539-541

DeGroot LJ, Larsen PR, Hennemann G. The thyroid and its diseases. 6th ed. New York: Churchill Livingston; 1996. p.659.

Department of Health Services, Radiation safety advisory 99-1, Subject: Probe-guided radiopharmaceuticals in the operating room. March 11,1999.

Doting MHE, Jansen L, Niegweg OE, et al. Lymphatic mapping with intralesional tracer administration in breast carcinoma patients. Cancer 2000;88(11):2546-2552

Ege GN. Lymphoscintigraphy--techniques and applications in the management of breast carcinoma. Seminars in Nuclear Medicine 1983;13(1):26-34

Ege GN. Internal mammary lymphoscintigraphy in breast carcinoma: a study of 1072 patients. International Journal of Radiation Oncology, Biology, Physics 1977;2(7-8):755-61

Eshima D, Eshima LA, Gotti NM, et al. Technetium-99m-sulfur colloid for lymphoscintigraphy: effects of preparation parameters. Journal of Nuclear Medicine 1996;37(9):1575-8

Fitzgibbons PL, LiVolsi VA, Surgical Pathology Committee of the College of American Pathologist, et al. Recommendations for handling radioactive specimens obtained by sentinel lymphadenectomy. American Journal of Surgical Pathology 2000;24(11):1549-51

Giuliano AE, Kirgan DM, Guenther JM, Morton DL. Lymphatic mapping and sentinel lymphadenectomy for breast cancer. Annals of Surgery 1994;220(3):391-8

Glass EC, Essner R, Morton DL. Kinetics of three lymphoscintigraphic agents in patients with cutaneous melanoma. Journal of Nuclear Medicine 1998;39(7):1185-90

Gould EA, Winship T, Philbin PH, Hyland KH. Observations on a "sentinel node" in cancer of the parotid. Cancer 1960:77-78

Grant RN, Tabah EJ, Adair FE. The surgical significance of the subareolar plexus in cancer of the breast. Surgery 1959;33:71-78

Gunter DL. Collimator characteristics and design. In: Henkin RE, et al, editors. Nuclear Medicine. St. Louis: Mosby; 1996. p.96-123.

Hill A, Tran K, Akhurst T, et al. Lessons learned from 500 cases of lymphatic mapping for breast cancer. Annals of Surgery 1999; 229:528-535

Hoffman EJ, Tornai MP, Janecek M, et al. Intraoperative probes and imaging probes. European Journal of Nuclear Medicine 1999;26(8):913-35

Klimberg VS, Rubio IT, Henry R, et al. Subareolar versus peritumoral injection for location of the sentinel lymph node. Annals of Surgery 1999;229(6):860-4; discussion 864-5

Kazem L, Antoniades J, Brady LW, et al. Clinical evaluation of lymph node scanning utilizing colloidal gold 198. Radiology 1968;90:905-911

Kowalsky RJ, Perry JR. Radiopharmaceuticals in Nuclear Medicine Practice. Norwalk:Appleton and Lange; 1987. p. 271-314.

Kern KA, Rosenberg RJ. Preroperataive lymphoscintigraphy during lymphatic mapping for breast cancer: improved sentinel node imaging using subareolar injection of technetium 99m sulfur colloid. Journal of the American College of Surgeons 2000;191(5):479-89

Krag D, Weaver D, Ashikaga T, et al. The sentinel node in breast cancer--a multicenter validation study. New England Journal of Medicine 1998;339(14):941-6

Krag DN, Meijer SJ, Weaver DL, et al. Minimal-access surgery for staging of malignant melanoma. Archives of Surgery 1995;130(6):654-8

Linehan DC, Hill ADK, Akhurst T, et al. Intradermal Radiocolloid and Intraparenchymal Blue Dye Injection Optimize Sentinel Node Identification in Breast Cancer Patients. Annals of Surgical Oncology 1999a;6(5):450-4

Linehan DC, Hill AD, Tran KN, et al. Sentinel lymph node biopsy in breast cancer: unfiltered radioisotope is superior to filtered. Journal of the American College of Surgeons 1999b;188(4):377-81

Miner TJ, Shriver CD, Jaques DP, et al. Ultrasonographically guided injection improves localization of radiolabeled sentinel node in breast cancer. Annals of Surgery 1998;5(6):315-21

Morita ET, Chang J, Leong SPL. Principles and controversies in lymphoscintigraphywith emphasis on breast cancer. In: Leong SPL, Wong JH, editors. Surgical Clinics of North America: Sentinel Lymph Nodes in Human Solid Cancer. Philadelphia: W. B. Saunders, 2000;80(6):1721-39

Morton DL, Chan AD. Current status of intraoperative lymphatic mapping and sentinel lymphadenectomy for melanoma: is it standard of care? Journal of the American College of Surgeons 1999a;189(2):214-23

Morton DL, Ollila DW. Critical review of the sentinel node hypothesis. Surgery 1999b;126(5):815-9

Morton DL. Intraoperative lymphatic mapping and sentinel lymphadenectomy: community standard care or clinical investigation? [comment]. Cancer Journal 1997a;3(6):328-30

Morton DL. Sentinel lymphadenectomy for patients with clinical stage I melanoma. Journal of Surgical Oncology 1997b;66(4):267-9

Morton DL, Wen DR, Cochran AJ. Management of early stage melanoma by intraoperative lymphatic mapping and selective lymphadenectomy. In: Coit DG, editor. Surgical Oncology Clinics of North America: Lymph Nodes Dissection in Malignant Melanoma. Philadelphia: WB Saunders, 1992a;1(2):247-59

Morton DL, Wen DR, Wong JH, et al. Technical details of intraoperative lymphatic mapping for early stage melanoma. Archives of Surgery 1992b;127(4):392-9

Porter GA, Ross MI, Berman RS, et al. How many lymph nodes are enough during sentinel lymphadenectomy for primary melanoma? Surgery 2000;128(2):306-11

Reintgen DS, Brobeil A. Lymphatic mapping and selective lymphadenectomy as an alternative to elective lymph node dissection in patients with malignant melanoma. Hematology/Oncology Clinics of North America 1998a;12(4):807-21, vii

Reintgen D, Cox C, Haddad F, et al. The role of lymphoscintigraphy in lymphatic mapping for melanoma and breast cancer [news]. Journal of Nuclear Medicine 1998b;39(12):22N, 25N, 32N, 36N

Reintgen D. Lymphatic mapping and sentinel node harvest for malignant melanoma. Journal of Surgical Oncology 1997;66(4):277-81

Russell JR, Stabin MG, Sparks RB, Watson E. Radiation absorbed dose to the embryo/fetus from radiopharmaceuticals. Health Physics 1997:73(5):756-69

Schneebaum S, Even-Sapir E, Cohen M, et al. Clinical applications of gamma-detection probes radioguided surgery. European Journal of Nuclear Medicine 1999;26(4 Suppl):S26-35

Simmons G. Gamma camera imaging systems. In: Henkin RE, et al, editors. Nuclear Medicine. St. Louis: Mosby; 1996. P.85-95.

Tonakie A, Sondak V, Yahanda A, Wahl RL. Reproducibility of lymphoscintigraphic drainage patterns in sequential Tc99m HSA and Tc99m sulfur colloid studies: implications for sentinel node identification in melanoma. Surgery 1999;126(5):955-962

Turner-Warwick RT. The lymphatics of the breast. British Journal of Surgery 1953;46:574-82

Vendrell-Torne E, Setoain-Quinquer J, Domenech-Torne FM. Study of normal mammary lymphatic drainage using radioactive isotopes. Journal of Nuclear Medicine 1972;13(11):801-5

Veronesi U, Paganelli G, Viale G, et al. Sentinel lymph node biopsy and axillary dissection in breast cancer: results in a large series. Journal of the National Cancer Institute 1999;91(4):368-373

Veronesi U, Pagannelli G, Galimberti V, et al. Sentinel node biopsy to avoid axillary dissection in breast cancer with clinically negative lymph nodes. Lancet 1997;349:1864-7

Uren RF, Howman-Giles RB, Thompson JF, et al. Mammary lymphoscintigraphy in breast cancer. Journal of Nuclear Medicine 1995;36(10):1775-80

Uren RF, Howman-Giles R, Thompson JF, et al.. Lymphatic drainage to the triangular intermuscular space lymph nodes in melanomas of the back. Journal of Nuclear Medicine 1996;37(6):964-6

Wong JH, Cagle LA, Morton DL. Lymphatic drainage of skin to sentinel lymph node in a feline model. Annals of Surgery 1991;214(5):637-41

Zanzonico P, Heller S. The intraoperative gamma probe: basic principles and choices available. Seminars in Nuclear Medicine 2000;30(1):33-48

3 SELECTIVE SENTINEL LYMPH NODE MAPPING AND DISSECTION FOR MALIGNANT MELANOMA

Stanley P. L. Leong, MD

RATIONALE FOR SELECTIVE SENTINEL LYMPHADENECTOMY FOR MELANOMA

Numerous retrospective studies have suggested that patients with primary melanoma who underwent elective lymph node dissection (ELND) had an improved survival rate as compared to patients who were initially observed and then underwent therapeutic lymph node dissection following the development of clinically evident regional metastasis [Balch 1981, Balch 1988, Callery 1982, Cohen 1977, Das Gupta 1977, McNeer 1964, Meyer 1979, Morton 1992a, Morton 1992b, Roses 1985]. ELND remains controversial despite a few prospectively randomized studies showed no notable benefit was obtained [Sim 1978, Veronesi 1977, Balch 1996, Balch 2000]. However, subgroup analysis in the study by Balch, et al. [1996, 2000] suggested that ELND may improve survival for male patients with lesions measuring 1.1 to 2 mm thick and 60 years of age or younger. As the incidence of microscopic metastasis in the prospective collection of patients with intermediate-thickness melanoma is approximately 20% [Morton 1992b] and because improvement in 5-year survival by ELND is approximately 53% versus about 26% following therapeutic dissection for palpable metastasis [Morton 1992b], ELND may be expected to influence the survival of less than 10% of the patients undergoing the procedure [Karakousis 1996a]. This may explain the difficulty in demonstrating survival benefit in prospective, randomized studies. Because most patients with primary melanoma do not harbor nodal metastases, they probably will not benefit from ELND, and yet ELND can result in postoperative limb edema. On the other hand, delay of ELND until the presence of palpable nodes may allow the spread of melanoma to other nodes and distant sites with a marked compromise of long-term survival. Sentinel lymph node (SLN) detection solves the clinical dilemma of selecting out the relevant node in the nodal basin. It is an ideal procedure because it is minimally invasive, yet powerful enough to select the relevant lymph node of the nodal basin, without a complete radical lymph node dissection. Another advantage of the SLN technique is that because significantly fewer lymph nodes are harvested, the harvested nodes can be processed meticulously to look for occult micrometastasis. Selective SLN dissection provides a suitable alternative to ELND in assessing patients with primary melanoma for the occurrence of microscopic metastasis.

IDENTIFICATION OF SLNs BY BLUE DYE VERSUS RADIOISOTOPE TECHNIQUE

Intraoperative localization of the SLN is accomplished by injection of two tracer agents at the primary site: Technetium-99m sulfur colloid and Lymphazurin or blue dye. This technique is based on the observation that when a blue dye such as isosulfan blue (Lymphazurin, Hirsch Industries, Inc., Richmond, VA) is injected around the primary melanoma site, it drains into the SLN. If the blue dye-stained SLN is negative for metastatic melanoma, then the incidence of micrometastasis in the remaining lymph node basin is less than 1%-2% [Morton 1992b]. Therefore, it can be concluded that the SLNs are the primary recipients of metastatic cells in most patients. When only using blue dye to find the SLNs, the dissection procedure could be relatively extensive. Injection of a radiocolloid at the primary melanoma site for lymphoscintigraphy has been used since the late 1970's [Fee 1978, Lamki 1992, Sullivan 1981] to guide surgeons for prophylactic lymph node dissection. Similar to blue dye, the radiocolloid enters lymphatic capillaries and concentrates in the SLNs. As shown by Alex and Krag [Alex 1993], a small hand-held gamma probe can be used to localize the radiolabeled lymph node in the regional nodal basin. Preoperative lymphoscintigraphy is also important because it defines the SLN from the primary site and it directs the surgical incisions. With the combination of blue dye and radioisotope mapping, the SLNs can be harvested with a minimal amount of dissection. A summary of the numerous studies using blue dye technique, radiotracer mapping by a hand-held gamma probe, or a combination of both techniques is shown in Table 1. Overall, the success rate of harvesting the SLN by blue dye alone is 82%, by radiotracer mapping is 94%, and by combination method is 98%. When SLNs by blue dye staining and/or are negative for micrometastasis, the remainder of the lymph node basin is usually negative [Morton 1992b, Reintgen 1994, Albertini 1996, Krag 1995, Ross 1993, Thompson 1994].

Different types of radiocolloid have been used such as Tc99m sulfur colloid with human serum albumin, Tc99m antimony sulfur colloid, and Tc99m sulfur colloid for identification of SLNs [Eshima 2000]. The ideal radioisotope colloid is one that, after injection, moves rapidly to the regional lymph node and concentrates in that node without leakage for at least several hours. This allows the patient to be transported to the operating room within a reasonable period of time for successful intraoperative mapping using a hand-held gamma probe without contaminating the rest of the nodal basin. Based on the studies by Albertini et al. [1996], the Tc99m sulfur colloid has been shown to concentrate in the regional lymph node within at least 3-6 hours. Comparisons have been made between the radioactivity of the SLN being harvested immediately following injection of the radiocolloid material and after 3-4 hours of injection. The radioactivity of the delayed SLN (n=16) was much higher than that of the immediate group (n=90) (p<0.01). This result indicated that Tc99m on injection would migrate quickly to the SLN and concentrate within it for at least 4 hours without significant leakage. In our study, this phenomenon of sustained concentration of radioisotope in the SLN has been substantiated. The average time of imaging between radiocolloid injection and lymph node identification by lymphoscintigraphy was 55 minutes (range 1-165 minutes) and an additional delay of 139 minutes (range 60-413 minutes) to the time of surgery. Furthermore, we have demonstrated that Tc99m

Table 1. Success Rates of Melanoma Sentinel Lymph Node Identification Techniques*

Author	Year	Patients	Blue Dye Technique	Intraoperative Radiotracer Technique	Either Technique
Morton [1992b]	1992	223	82% (basins)	not used	
Reintgen [1994]	1994	42	100% (patients)	not used	
Van der Veen [1994]	1994	11	100% (patients)	100% (patients)	
Glass [1995]	1995	132	99% (patients)	not indicated	100% (patients)
Krag [1995]	1995	121	91% (patients)	98% (patients)	
Pijpers [1995]	1995	41	90% (patients)	100% patients	
Glass [1996]	1996	148	60% (nodes)	80% (nodes)	97% (nodes)
Karakousis [1996b]	1996	55	93% (patients)	not used	
Albertini [1996]	1996	106	70% (nodes)	84% (nodes)	96% (basins)
Kapteijn [1997]	1997	110	84% (nodes)	99.5% (nodes)	99.5% (nodes)
Leong [1997]	1997	163	74% (nodes)	98% (nodes)	
Bostick [1997]	1997	117	92% (basins)	100% (basins)	100% (basins)
Pijpers [1997]	1997	135	86% (nodes) 85% (basins)	100% (nodes) 100% (basins)	
Wells [1997]	1997	58	67% (nodes)	not indicated	95% (patients)
Lingam [1997]	1997	35	100% (patients)	not used	
Joseph [1997]	1997	595	not indicated	not indicated	98% (patients)

* Reporting of success rates is not standardized. Percentages are indicated in patients, nodal basins or SLNs. Furthermore, common denominators, such as total number of SLND attempts, are not always explicitly mentioned. Thus, the above percentages may vary depending on interpretation. From Leong, SPL: The role of sentinel lymph nodes in human solid cancer. In: Devita, VT, Hellman, S, Rosenberg, SA, eds. PPO Updates, vol 12., Philadelphia: Lippincott-Raven, 1998; with permission.

can be detected in SLNs up to nearly 7 hours without significant leakage of the radioisotope to the adjacent lymph nodes nor the adjacent lymphatic tissue. We have imaged over 20 patients at delayed times over 18 hours, but have not seen further migration to other sites (data not shown).

In comparing the two techniques, gamma probe lymphoscintigraphy has been seen to be superior to blue dye in the detection of SLNs. Following Lymphazurin injection, blue dye-stained lymphatics and lymph nodes could easily be visualized in 74.1% of the SLNs. When radiocolloid was used to locate SLNs, a SLN was defined as any lymph node with radioactivity greater than three times the background *in vivo* or 10 times the background *ex vivo* [Albertini 1996]. Using this definition, 98% of the cases of SLNs were determined using the gamma probe. In about 30% of the cases, no blue lymphatics were seen. In such cases, gamma probe detection was crucial in detecting the SLNs.

The stable accumulation of the Tc99m in the SLNs for several hours allows us to admit the patient, and perform preoperative lymphoscintigraphy, intraoperative mapping, and surgery all on the same day. This eliminates the necessity of the surgeon injecting radioisotope material in the operating room. In our study, as well as in other studies [Albertini 1996, Krag 1995, Reintgen 1994, Ross 1993, Thompson 1994], the successful identification and harvesting of SLN is high, approaching more than 95%. A recent study has demonstrated no significant discordancy between immediate and overnight patterns of lymphoscintigraphy [White 1999]. We have performed over 20 cases on patients with extremity melanoma. Lymphoscintigraphy on the day before and the next day prior to surgery showed a concordancy rate of almost 100% (unpublished data). Therefore, patients, certainly those with melanoma of the extremity, may have preoperative lymphoscintigraphy the night before surgery and can be scheduled for the first case the next day without delay in the nuclear medicine suite.

As the radioisotope accumulates in the SLN following preoperative lymphoscintigraphy, the patient can be immediately transferred to the operating room for intraoperative mapping with blue dye injection as well as with a hand-held gamma probe. We have taken advantage of this approach and streamlined the patient's initial preoperative lymphoscintigraphy and intraoperative mapping within the same day of surgery, to avoid two different injections of radioisotope and a separate lymphoscintigraphy prior to surgery [Leong 1997].

SELECTIVE SENTINEL LYMPH NODE MAPPING FOR MELANOMA: HOW WE DO IT

I. Preoperative Lymphoscintigraphy
The use of the gamma camera to localize the SLN is important although Krag states that imaging is not necessary [Krag 1998]. At UCSF Medical Center at Mount Zion, we have developed a close working relationship between the nuclear medicine physician and the surgical staff. The imaging information is communicated to the surgeon prior to selective SLN dissection. This practice gives the surgeon a greater confidence in localizing the lymph node. In-transit nodes and other basins for consideration are noted. Although Krag has defined nodes with ease using the gamma probe alone, we consider imaging with associated marks on the patient's skin to limit the time of search and the size of the incision for the SLN.

Preparation of Tc99m Sulfur Colloid
The sulfur colloid is made by a hydrogen sulfide technique [Kowalsky 1987], which makes the particles much smaller than the standard thiosulfate method [Kowalsky 1987]. The radiocolloid is filtered through a 22-μm filter to remove any large particles.

Injection of Sulfur Colloid
The average injected dose of Tc99m in our series of patients was 20.7 MBg (range, 3.7-74 MBg). The time from radioisotope injection to surgical incision ranged from 60 to 413 minutes (mean time, 139 min.).

Identification of Lymphatic Basins
Lymphatic basins at risk are identified by the nuclear medicine physician, and the location of the highest radioisotope uptake is marked to indicate the presence of the SLN in each of the basins. In most of the cases the lymphatic channels are

visualized leading to the SLN. We have learned that it may be necessary to cover the injection site with lead to visualize the lymphatic channels, especially if the injection site is in the field of view with the SLN such as in head and neck sites. Figure 1 (pg. 47) shows the different possible patterns of channels leading to the SLNs. For more detailed information, see Chapter 2.

II. Intraoperative Mapping Technique
Lymphazurin Injection
After the SLN site is marked, the patient is transferred to the operating room. No further injection of radiotracer is necessary in the operating room. Lymphazurin is injected intradermally prior to the procedure around the primary melanoma site ranging from 1 to 5 ml. The surgical wounds are then prepared. Be aware of any adverse reactions such as urticaria, respiratory and hemodynamic changes which usually occur in the first 10 to 20 minutes. [Leong 2000b]. The patient should be instructed that his or her urine will be blue for several days, as the blue dye also enters the circulatory system.

Types of Anesthesia
General anesthesia has been used preferentially (77.5%), as compared to monitored anesthesia care (17.2%), regional (4.6%) and local (0.7%).

Intraoperative Mapping
Intraoperative mapping of the SLNs is achieved using a hand-held gamma probe (Neoprobe 2000, Neoprobe Corporation. Dublin, OH) and staining with blue dye. A 2-3 cm incision is made over the marked area of greatest activity as detected by the hand-held gamma probe. The incision is carried down through the subcutaneous fat in a tunnel-like fashion, and the fascia is incised. The lymph nodes usually reside beneath the fascia. Using the gamma probe, the SLNs can be located by detecting increased radioactivity in counts per second with respect to orientation. Often, the blue dye-stained lymphatics would be seen, confirming the findings of the radioisotope activity, with resultant removal of the SLN. Always proceed the dissection as close to the SLN as possible to avoid injury to nerves and vessels. In general, the SLN may be identified using a gamma probe, blue dye, or both.

Identification of SLNs
After the removal of the SLN, the hand-held gamma probe is used to search the resection bed to make sure that no residual elevated radioactivity remained. Further exploration is carried out, if the resection bed count remained high. Figures 2 and 3 (pg. 48) show two patterns of resection bed radioactivity, as determined by a gamma probe, depending on the number of SLNs. If only one SLN is present, the resection bed count is almost equal to background levels. On the other hand, when multiple SLNs are present, the resection bed, after removal of the first SLN, shows persistent elevation of radioactivity until the last SLN is removed, at which time there is a decrease in the resection bed count to almost background levels (Figure 3, pg. 48). In general, the presence of residual SLNs in the basin should be considered if the resection bed-to-background ratio remains above 3:1 or if the node shows an

in situ count >10% hottest node. The author always does a "roaming count" at 8 positions of the clock to make sure the entire operative field is of low background count. Roaming and resection bed counts should be carefully taken. The resection bed count is the count where the lymph node has been harvested and therefore it should be to normal background or at least significantly drops down unless there is an adjacent "hot" lymph node. On the other hand, roaming counts may be elevated despite the fact that the resection bed count is low because an elevated roaming count wherever that elevation is indicates a separate SLN. Prior to closure, a digital exploration is also important to make sure that no suspicious nodes are left behind. When a SLN is totally replaced by tumor cells, it may not pick up the blue dye or radiocolloid, presumably due to blockage of the tracer from entering into the lymph node.

Advantage of the Gamma Probe
The intraoperative hand-held gamma probe directs the surgeon to the area of greatest radioactivity with pinpoint accuracy. This often results in the identification of blue dye-stained lymphatics that otherwise would require a more extensive dissection to detect. The radiolabeled lymph nodes could be easily detected using a hand-held gamma probe [Alex 1993]. Therefore, with the combination of the blue dye and radioisotope mapping, the SLNs can be harvested with minimal extent of dissection [Krag 1995, Albertini 1996, Kapteijn 1997, Leong 1997, Bostick 1997, Pijpers 1997] and accuracy [Krag 1995, Morton 1992b, Reintgen 1994, Ross 1993, Thompson 1995]. The ability to visualize the afferent lymphatics and the lymph node with blue dye gives the surgeon the added dimension of direct identification of the lymph nodes, in addition to mapping by the gamma probe. In general, the primary melanoma site would be widely excised. Therefore, retention of the blue dye in the original melanoma or biopsy site is not a problem. Furthermore, the dye will dissipate in weeks if, indeed, there is some residual dye still left in the skin following wide excision. On average, the colloid or the blue dye will travel through the lymphatics to the appropriate SLNs within 5-15 minutes. For the group of patients almost 20% with no visible blue dye, the SLN exploration would have been unsuccessful if the gamma probe were not used.

Closure of Wounds
After selective SLN dissection, the wound is then closed in three layers, with the deep layer being closed with interrupted 2-0 Dexon (Davis & Geek Manati, PR) sutures, the superficial subcutaneous layer with interrupted 3-0 Dexon sutures, and the skin with either running subcuticular sutures of 4-0 Dexon. Particularly in the axilla, avoid placement of too deep a suture as nerves may be ligated. Drains are not placed. After changing gloves and instruments, the primary site is excised according to the thickness of the primary melanoma. Most of the time, the wound is closed primarily, and only occasionally are split-thickness skin grafts used. Complications of selective SLN dissection have been minor, and most patients have been discharged from the hospital either on the day of surgery or the day after.

Table Dissection

It is important to dissect the SLN from the non-SLN or lymphatic tissue within the resected specimen on a separate table using the gamma probe so that each lymph node is correctly labeled for pathologic evaluation.

III. Instruments

The author finds that several instruments (Figure 4, pg. 49) are indispensable for the successful performance of selective sentinel lymphadenectomy. The Baily right angle is a fine instrument for dividing the fascia from the subcutaneous tissue such as clavipectoral fascia in the axilla and Scarpa's fascia in the groin. A fine Schmidt clamp may also be used. Usually, the lymph nodes are situated beneath the fascia. The Allis clamp is routinely used to grasp the adjacent tissue surrounding the SLN to lift it from deep into the operative field. Alternatively a 2-0 silk stitch may serve the same purpose. The author finds that the Allis clamp is much more reliable. Since the incision is usually small 2-3 cm, three directional retraction is critical to expose the deeply seated SLN. Depending on the depth of the operative field, a vein retractor, Army and Navy, McBurney or Deaver retractor may be used.

IV. Case Illustrations

Several selected cases have been chosen from the author's extensive experience on melanoma selective sentinel lymphadenectomy. They are classified under head and neck (Figure 5, pg. 51), trunk (Figures 6, pg. 52 and 7, pg. 53) and extremities (Figures 8, pg. 54 and 9, pg.55). A sample operative report is included as an illustration of how the author dictates his operative report (Figure 10, pg. 56 and 57).

EMPHASIS FOR PREOPERTIVE LYMPHOSCINTIGRAPHY AND NARROW EXCISION OF SUSPECTED SKIN LESION FOR MELANOMA

Our recent study has found that discordancy between lymphoscintigraphic and clinically defined nodal basins is 5% for lower extremity, 14% for upper extremity, 25% for trunkal melanoma and 48% for head and neck. The overall discordancy rate is 19.5% [Leong 1999a]. Because of discordance between clinical predictions and lymphatic drainage as determined by preoperative lymphoscintigraphy [Leong 1999a] preoperative lymphoscintigraphy is a prerequisite for characterizing the lymphatic drainage pattern in patients with primary melanoma especially for sites such as the head and neck as well as the trunk before selective SLN dissection [Leong 1999a]. Our studies are in agreement with other studies [Wanebo 1985, Uren 1993, Berman 1992, Thompson 1994]. Therefore, it is mandatory to have preoperative lymphoscintigraphy prior to selective sentinel lymphadenectomy. Because of potential lymphatic drainage disruption by wide local re-excision, it is preferred to have re-excision performed in the same setting as the selective lymphadenectomy. For the sake of argument even if no disruptions were made by initial wide local re-excisions, concideration should be given to the patient so that re-excision can be done at the same time of selective sentinel lymphadenectomy [Coldiron 2000, Leong 2000e].

Therefore it is important to have a narrow biopsy of any suspected pigment liaison without a wide local excision. If the histological diagnosis is confirmed to be melanoma and fits the criteria for the selective sentinel lymphadenectomy such as Breslow thickness greater than 1 millimeters, transection of the melanoma without definitive thickness, regression and ulceration, wide local re-excision should be delayed until the time of sentinel lymphadenectomy.

CHOICE OF BLUE DYE VERSUS RADIOTRACER IN MAPPING THE SLN

Whether the choice of SLN localization method either by radioactivity or blue dye is of any clinical significance is undetermined at this time. However, 27.3% of the SLNs were detected using only the hand-held gamma probe with no blue dye staining [Leong 1997]. Some radiolabelled lymph nodes were positive for micrometastasis, certainly qualifying them as SLNs. Therefore, radiocolloid detection is more sensitive than the blue dye as shown in our study [Leong 1997] as well as in another study [Kapteijn 1997].

Our goal in this study was to correlate all the SLNs with metastatic melanoma with blue dye or radiotracer staining. Currently, the SLN is arbitrarily defined as a node that grossly harbors blue dye and/or shows radioactive uptake exceeding a 10:1 ratio of *ex vivo* to resection bed count or a 3:1 ratio of *in vivo* to resection bed count [Albertini 1996]. Our study included 309 consecutive patients who underwent melanoma SLN mapping procedure. Five hundred seventy seven lymph nodes were studied for blue dye intensity, radioactive uptake (hot) and presence of blue afferent lymphatic channels. In analysis, 54 of the 309 patients (17.5%) were found to have SLNs positive for melanoma, and 68 of the 577 SLNs harvested (11.8%) were found to harbor micrometastasis. The distribution of blue and hot SLNs positive for micrometastasis is summarized in Table 2.

Table 2. Distributions of Positive SLNs with respect to blue and "hot" nodes.

Positive SLNs by Tracer Identification	Number	Percentage
Blue Only	1	1.5
Blue and Hot	54	79.4
Hot Only	13	19.1
Total	68	100.0

Blue afferent lymphatic channels were not consistent in leading to a blue lymph node. For all the positive SLNs, the lowest *ex vivo* to resection bed count ratio exceeded a 3:1 ratio. Using positive SLNs as relevant references, almost all SLNs (98.5%) could be detected by increased radioactive uptake and yet only approximately 80.9% were visualized as blue. Furthermore, about 1% of the patients receiving blue dye manifested a severe anaphylactic reaction [Leong 2000b]. Therefore, we conclude that radioactive localization of SLN using gamma probe is a far superior technique than blue dye, and that in most cases, the radiotracer can replace the blue dye [Leong 2000d].

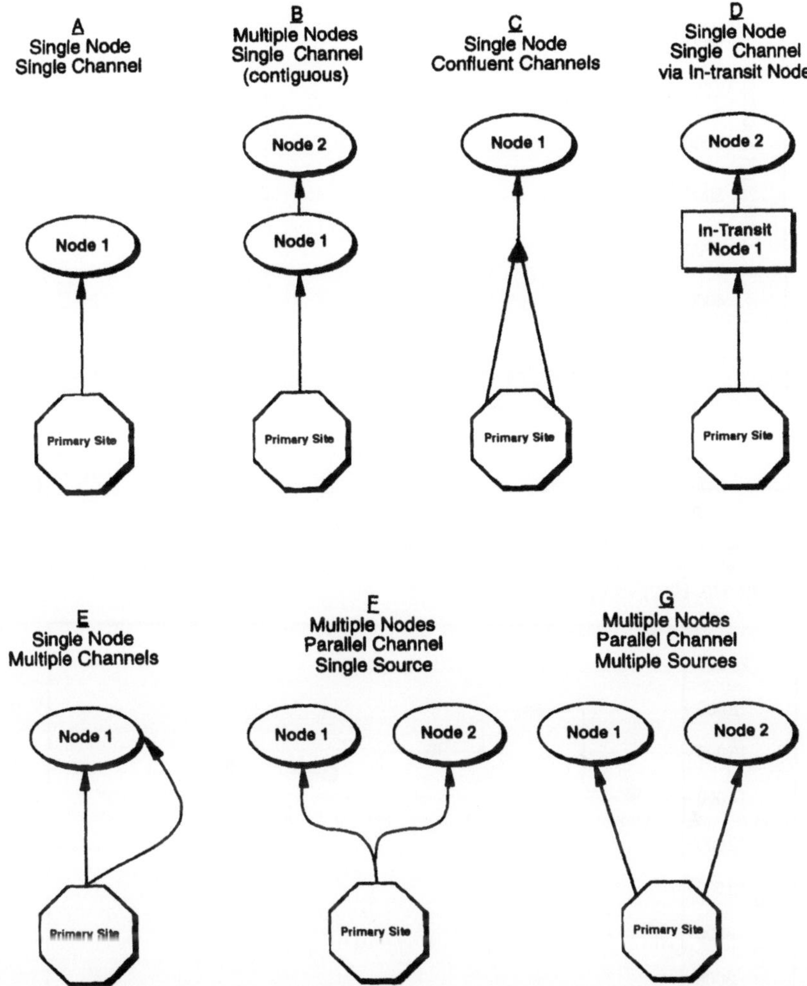

Figure 1. Different patterns of lymphatic channel between the primary site of melanoma and SLNs. Pattern A appears to be most frequent. Patterns C and E show two channels leading to one SLN. Pattern D shows occasional uptake of radioactivity in in-transit lymph nodes prior to the SLN in the regional lymph node basin. To date, both the in-transit lymph node and SLN are being biopsied when the in-transit lymph node is encountered. When a channel drains into a lymph node and contiguous to another lymph node in succession (Pattern B), the first lymph node is considered the SLN. On the other hand, when parallel channels are observed (Pattern F and G), both SLNs should be harvested. Further study is underway to identify the frequency of these different patterns of drainage to the regional SLNs. From Leong, SPL: The role of sentinel lymph nodes in human solid cancer. In: Devita, VT, Hellman, S, Rosenberg, SA, eds. PPO Updates, vol 12., Philadelphia: Lippincott-Raven, 1998; with permission.

                              Atlas of Selective Sentinel Lymphadenectomy

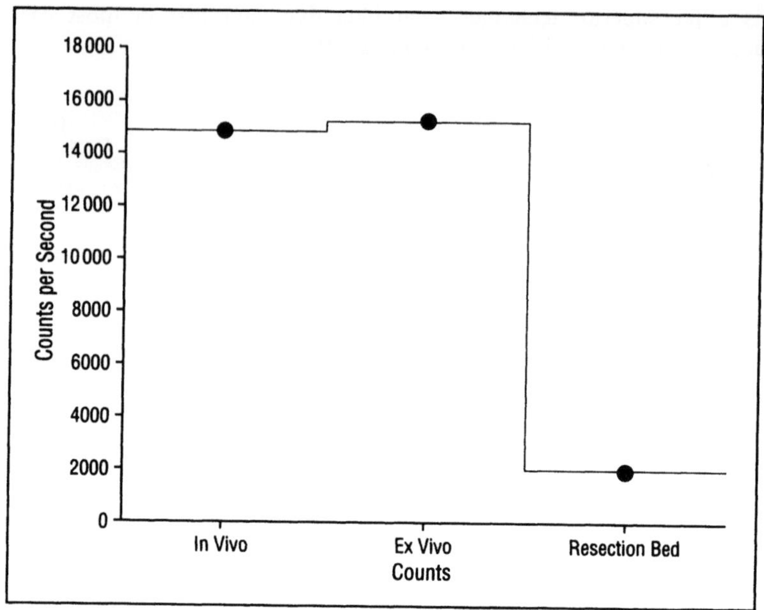

Figure 2. Pattern of radioactive counts per second in identifying a single SLN. After successful resection of the SLN, the resection bed counts returned to the background level. From Leong SPL, Steinmetz I, et al.: Optimal Selective Sentinel Lymph Node Dissection in Primary Malignant Melanoma. Arch Surg 132:670, 1997; with permission.

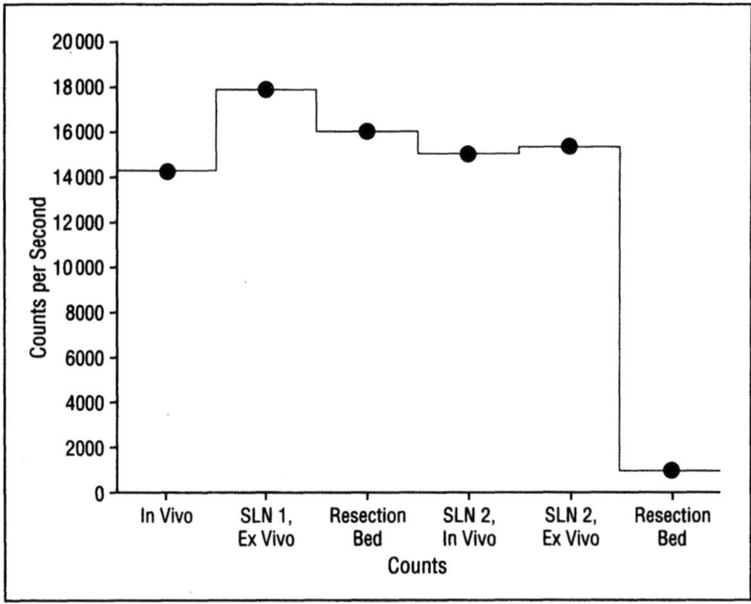

Figure 3. Pattern of radioactive counts per second in identifying multiple SLNs. After resection of the first SLN, the resection counts persisted to be high. When the second and last SLN was successfully resected, the resection bed counts returned to the background level. From Leong SPL, Steinmetz I, et al.: Optimal Selective Sentinel Lymph Node Dissection in Primary Malignant Melanoma. Arch Surg 132:670, 1997; with permission.

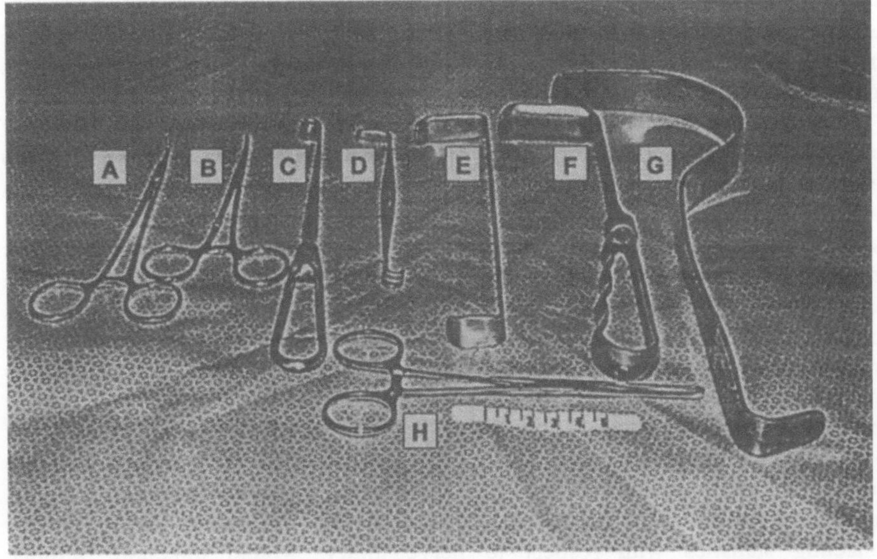

Figure 4. Instruments for selective sentinel lymphadenectomy:
A - Right Angle Bailey Clamp
B - Fine Schnidt Clamp
C - Vein Hook Retractor
D - Dull Senn Retractor
E - Army-Navy Retractor
F - McBurney Retractor
G - Deaver Retractor
H - Allis Clamp

COMPLICATIONS

We have reported severe anaphylactic reactions from blue dye [Leong 2000b]. From November, 1993 to August, 1998, 406 patients underwent intraoperative lymphatic mapping using both isosulfan blue (1-5cc injected intradermally around the primary melanoma) and radiocolloid injection at UCSF Medical Center at Mount Zion. Three cases of anaphylaxis following intradermal injection with isosulfan blue were encountered. These cases varied in severity from treatable hypotension with urticaria and erythema to severe cardiovascular collapse with or without bronchospasm or urticaria. In our series, the incidence of anaphylaxis to isosulfan blue was about 1%. Anaphylaxis can be fatal if not recognized and treated rapidly. Operating room personnel participating in intraoperative lymphatic mapping where isosulfan blue is used must be aware of the potential consequences and be prepared to treat anaphylaxis.

Recently Krouse and Schwarz in their letter to the ediitor of Annals of Surgical Oncology entitled *"Blue dye for sentinel lymph node mapping: not too sensitive, but too hypersensitive?,"* they described a case in which a melanoma patient following blue dye injection developed blue hives [Krouse 2000]. They assert that the utility of the routine use of blue dye for intraoperative mapping is probably not needed when a radiolabled SLN technique is to be performed. The author agrees with their suggestion [Leong 2000c]. The surgical and anesthesia complications of selective sentinel lymphadenectomy are consistant to the procedure performed. A recent study by Bonenkanp et al of 43 melanoma patients undergoing selective sentinel lymph node dissection show one of the axillary procedures was complicated by wound dehiscence (mobility 4%), and 4 of the 12 (30%) inguinal procedures were complicated by lymphocele or infection with one wound. Sentinel lymph node dissection in the neck region had no morbidity. All these complications were treated out of the hospital [Bonenkanp 2001]. We are collecting statistics with respect to nerve injury, wound infection, seroma, lymphaderma and so forth in a prospective fashion.

CLINICAL SIGNIFICANCE OF MELANOMA MICROMETASTASIS TO SENTINEL LYMPH NODES AND OTHER HIGH RISK FACTORS

According to recent studies by Gershenwald [Gershenwald 1999] and our group [Leong 2000a], patients with positive SLNs do much worse than those with negative SLNs with respect to disease-free survival. More than 600 patients who underwent lymphatic mapping at the M.D. Anderson Cancer Center and the University of South Florida were followed with a median follow-up of 20 months. The SLN status was analyzed using multivaried analysis in comparison to the other prognostic factors influencing the outcome of melanoma. SLN status was found to be the most important prognostic factor influencing disease-free and distal disease-free survival in stage I and II patients (p<0.02). Patients who had negative SLNs by

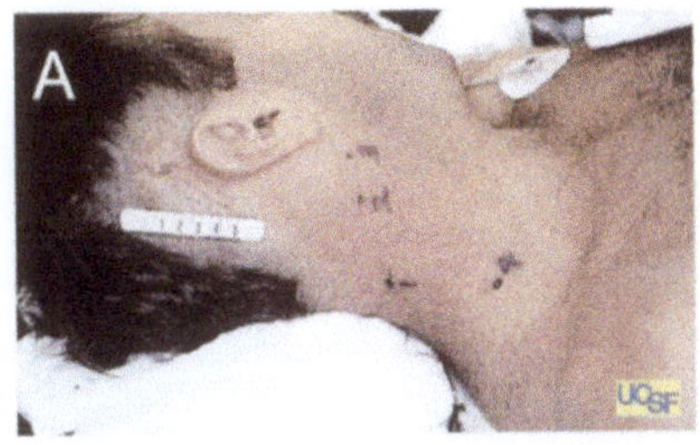
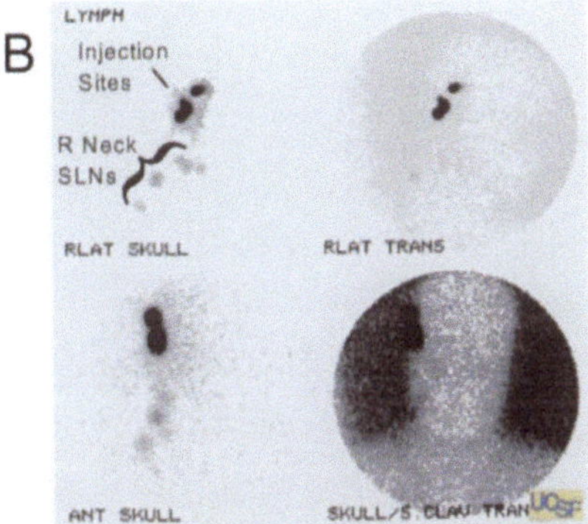

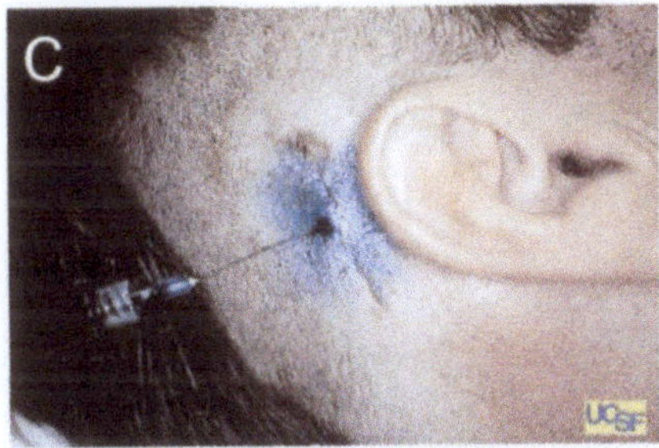
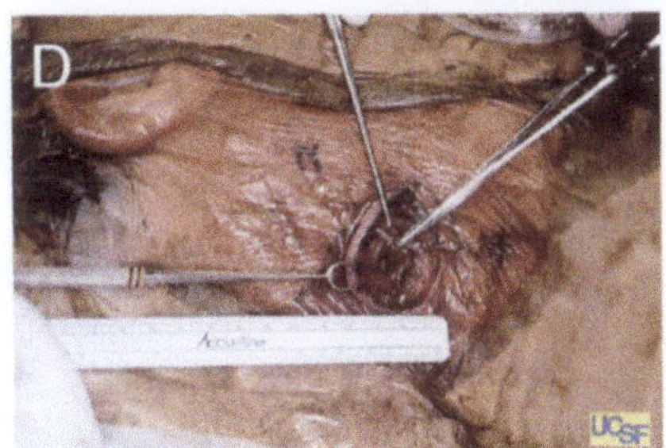

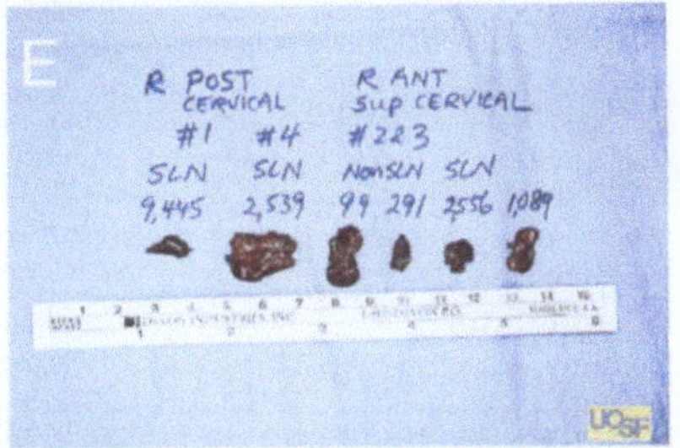

Figure 5 - Head and Neck

A 43 year old Caucasian male with melanoma of the right posterior auricular scalp area with a previous narrow biopsy showing Breslow thickness of 2.6mm, (Clark's level IV). His preoperative chest x-rays and blood tests were unremarkable. Preoperative lymphoscintigraphy revealed four areas of focal uptake consistent with nodal uptake in the right posterior cervical chains. Intraoperative mapping with intradermal injection of Isosulfan blue dye and gamma probe resulted in harvesting of several sentinel lymph nodes which were all negative for microscopic disease.

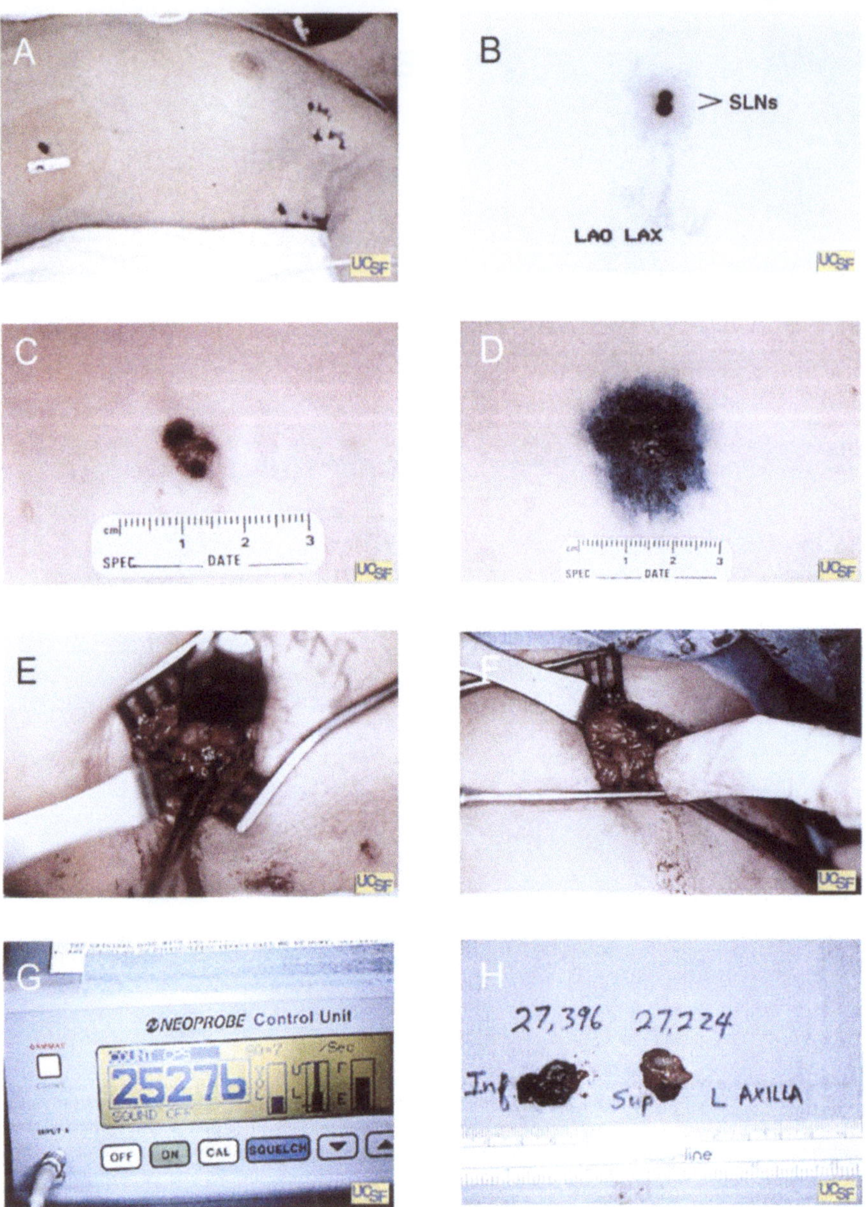

Figure 6 - Trunk

A 34 year old Caucasian female, presented with an abnormal changing mole in the left flank area. Partial punch biopsy of the lesion revealed malignant melanoma of 1.2 mm Breslow thickness (Clark's level III/IV). Preoperative chest x-rays and blood tests were unremarkable. Preoperative lymphoscintigraphy revealed two sentinel lymph nodes with a single channel to the left axilla. Intraoperative lymphatic mapping with intradermal Isosulfan blue dye injection and a gamma probe was successful in harvesting two sentinel lymph nodes, the second being located inferiorly to the first. Both nodes were found to be negative for micrometastasis. The patient has been followed up on a regular basis with no evidence of disease for 3 years and 9 months at the last clinic visit..

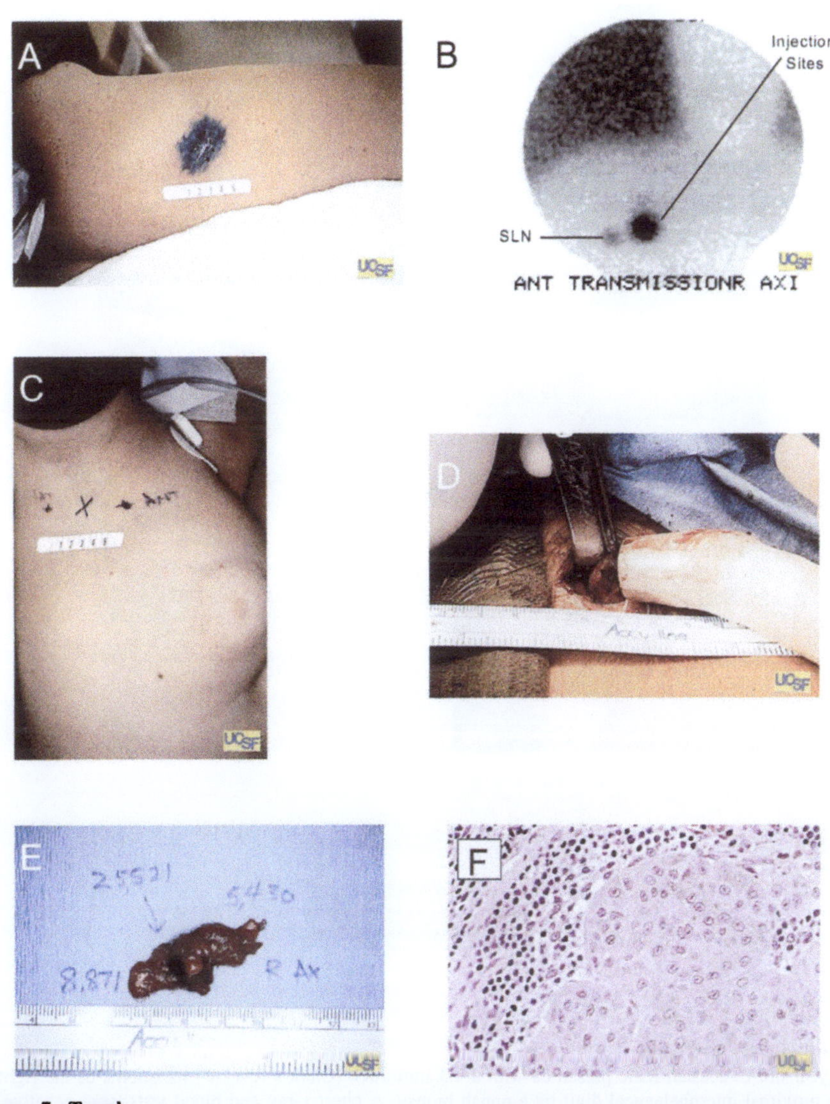

Figure 7 - Trunk
A 22 year old Caucasian female with a narrow biopsy of a changing mole in the right scapular area which revealed 1.3 mm Breslow thickness and an unclassified Clark's level. Her preoperative chest x-ray and blood tests were negative. Her preoperative lymphoscintigraphy showed a sentinel lymph node in the right axilla. Intraoperative lymphatic mapping including intradermal injection of Isosulfan blue dye and a gamma probe resulted in successful harvesting of a right axillary sentinel lymph node harboring micrometastasis. She subsequently underwent a negative right axillary level I/II/III radical lymph node dissection (0/15 nodes). She was subsequently treated with adjuvant Interferon for one year and has been free of disease for 3 1/2 years at the last clinic visit.

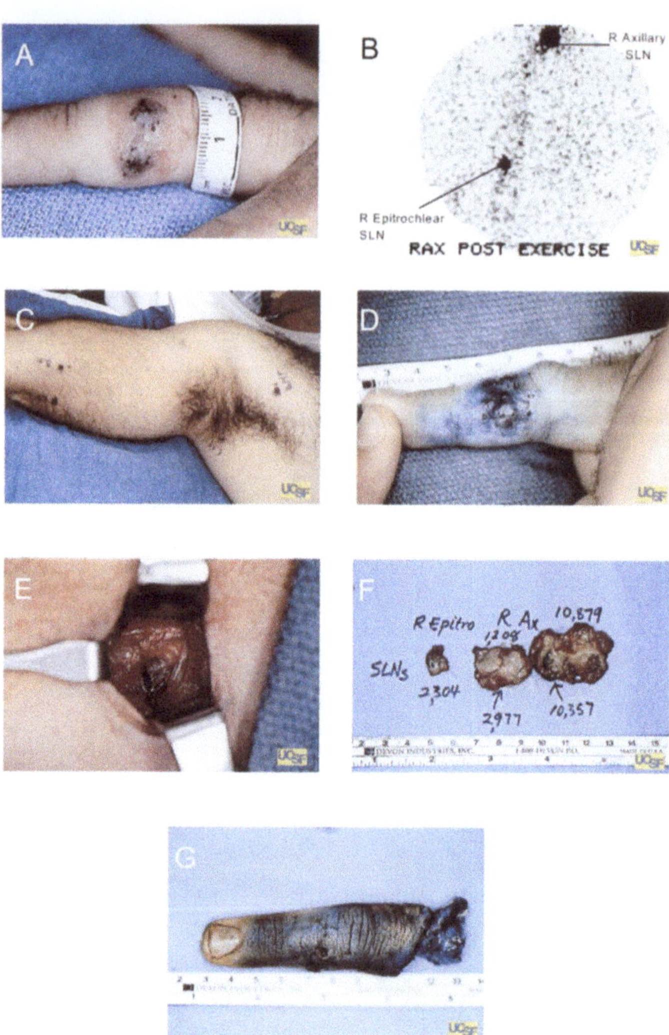

Figure 8 - Upper Extremity

A 37 year old Caucasian male presented with a 4.3 mm thick (Clark's level V) melanoma of the right fourth proximal interphalangeal digit by a punch biopsy. A chest x-ray and blood tests were negative. Preoperative lymphoscintigraphy revealed one lymph node in the right epitrochlear area and two in the right axilla. Intraoperative lymphatic mapping consisting of intradermal injection of Isosulfan blue dye and a gamma probe resulted in the successful harvesting of the sentinel nodes, all of which were found to be positive for micrometastasis. The primary lesion was found to have a thickness of 4.5 mm (Clark's level V). The patient also underwent amputation of the finger. His postoperative course was uneventful. As a member of a certain religious faith, the patient declined any subsequent treatment including additional lymph node dissection and interferon. He underwent alternative medical treatment. Four months following initial surgery, a lesion the size of a golf ball developed in the right preauricular area. Six months following initial surgery, he developed recurrence in the right axilla. There was no recurrence in the right epitrochlear area or at the amputation site. The patient ultimately expired one year later secondary to metastatic melanoma.

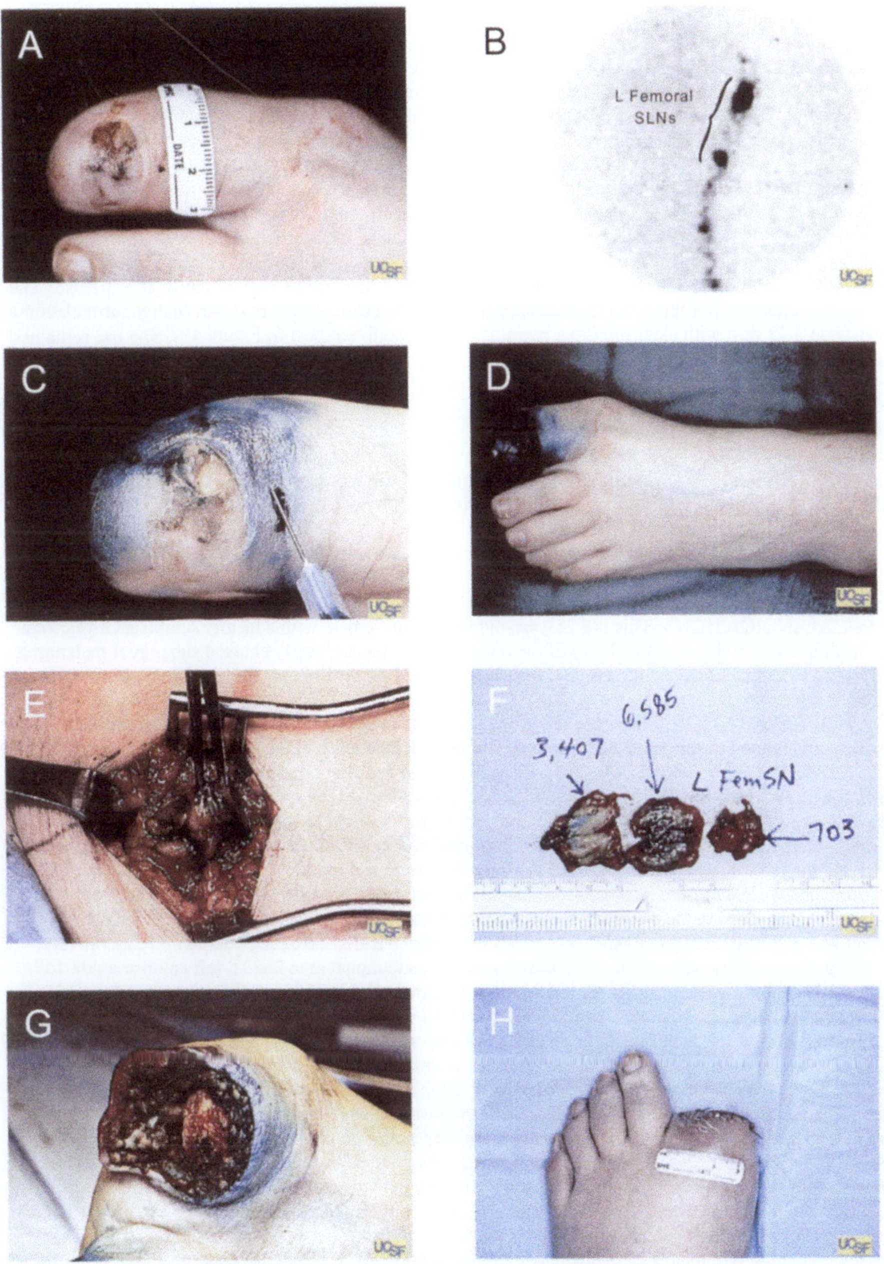

Figure 9 - Lower Extremity

A 78 year old Caucasian female presented with a history of a left great toe melanoma after some tissue was debrided for a nonhealing ulcer following local trauma the previous year. Biopsy was significant for an undifferentiated neoplasm consistent with melanoma. S-100 and HMB-45 stains were positive. The patient had no palpable lymphadenopathy. Her preoperative chest x-rays and blood tests were negative. Preoperative lymphoscintigraphy revealed a single channel leading to two prominent contiguous sentinel lymph nodes in the left superficial inguinal basin. However, the patient, who has a history of a stable angina, did not undergo subsequent surgery due to a cardiac assessment. Preoperative lymphoscintigraphy was performed again 1 week later and revealed the same sentinel lymph node pattern from the previous study. The sentinel nodes were marked. The more proximal of the "hot" areas showed the most intense activity. The distal one had lesser activity and the dynamic study actually intensified at a somewhat later time. It was commented in the lymphoscintigraphy report that this might be simply confluence of lymphatic vessels rather than a definite node, although this area was marked. The popliteal area was negative. Intraoperative lymphatic mapping including intradermal Isosulfan blue dye injection and a gamma probe resulted in successful harvesting of 2 SLNs and an distal adjacent lymphatic tissue in the left femoral area, which were all confirmed by Pathology to be free of metastatic disease. The patient also underwent a left great toe transphalangeal amputiation which revealed malignant melanoma invasive to 3.12 mm with clear proximal margins. (See operative report in Figure 10). She has remained disease free for 46 months as of her last clinic visit.

Patient Name: Patient from Figure 9   MRN: #
PREOPERATIVE DIAGNOSIS: Malignant melanoma of the subungual type of the left great toe.
POSTOPERATIVE DIAGNOSIS: Malignant melanoma of the subungual type of the left great toe.
OPERATION: 1. Left femoral selective sentinel lymph node dissection with intraoperative
                      lymphatic mapping.
                      2. Amputation of the left great toe at the proximal aspect of the proximal
                      phalangeal joint.
ANESTHESIA: Spinal anesthesia.
CLINICAL INDICATIONS: This is a 78-year-old Caucasian female with a history of at least a year of a non-healing ulcer in the subungual area of the left great toe. Recent biopsy showed subungual melanoma. She has no evidence of metastatic disease. She was admitted at this time for the procedures as mentioned below.
WOUND PREPARATION: The entire left lower extremity to above the left groin was painted with Betadine and draped in the usual sterile fashion with a stockinette up to the level of the midthigh.
DESCRIPTION OF PROCEDURE: The patient first underwent lymphscintigraphy in the Nuclear Medicine Department and 287 microcurie of technetium sulfur colloid were injected in the left subungual area at 9:00 am. One lymph node basin was noted in the left femoral triangle and two "hot" areas were marked - one proximally and one distally. The proximal marking was 3 cm below the inguinal crease overlying the femoral artery and the distal marking was distal and medial to the proximal marking at 7.5 cm from the inguinal crease. Informed consent was signed. I was present throughout the entire procedure. The patient was taken to the operating room and satisfactory spinal anesthesia was performed. The patient was placed in the supine position with the left knee in a slight frog leg position. Preoperatively, the Neoprobe readings were taken of the primary site left subungual area 26232, left anterior ankle 157, popliteal 37, left midanterior thigh 77, left femoral proximal marking 3898, left femoral distal marking 507, a point between the two markings 573, left proximal inguinal 906, suprapubic 471, right femoral (the contralateral to the proximal marking of the left femoral triangle) 102, right femoral (contralateral to the distal marking of the left femoral area) 155, and umbilicus 164.
The patient received 1 gm of Kefzol preoperatively. Blue dye injection was given at 14:15 and blue dye injection was completed at about 14:29. 5 cc* of Lymphazurin were injected around the left subungual area in a circumferential way. Blue lymphatics were seen going up the dorsal surface of the left foot towards the ankle. An incision was made at 14:46 of a distance of about 3 cm just below the proximal marking along the axis of the left femoral artery. The incision was carried through the Scarpa's fascia. At 2 cm below the incision at 14:52 proximal pointing, the count was 5217. At 14:54, at 3 cm below the skin level, proximal pointing the reading was 6001. At 14:55, the blue lymphatics were scored as 4/5.
At 15:12, the blue lymphatics were noted to be draining into two lymph nodes underneath the proximal marking and there were two lymph nodes - one proximally and the other distally located as a chain of two lymph nodes. The reading on the proximal lymph node was 4663 and that of the distal lymph node which was larger than the proximal lymph node was 6601. The proximal lymph node was 3/5 blue and the distal lymph node was also 3/5 blue. Lymph nodes were secured with an Allis clamp and dissected from the surrounding tissue using hemoclips to clip the lymphatic tissue. At 15:13, both lymph nodes were removed and the ex vivo reading of the proximal lymph node was 3729 and the distal lymph node was 6474. At 15:15, the surgical bed was 367. The roaming counts proximally 752, superolaterally 251, laterally 131, inferolaterally 74, distally 92, inferomedially 152, medially 91, superomedially 348.

Because there was a distal marking; a distal flap was created to dissect to the distal marking area and the readings were from 95-192; therefore, it was thought that the distal marking did not represent a true lymph node underneath. Digital exploration showed no residual suspicious or enlarged lymph nodes in the surgical bed. The wound was irrigated with saline and the deep subcutaneous layer was closed with interrupted stitches of 3-0 Dexon. The superficial subcutaneous layer was also closed with interrupted stitches of 3-0 Dexon. The skin was closed with running subcuticular stitches of 4-0 Dexon. Instruments and gloves were all changed. Attention was then directed towards the left great toe. This was approached by removing the drapes and underneath it was isolated clean drapes as well as the stockinette. The stockinette was then cut and this exposed the left great toe. The left great toe was wrapped around with a 4x4 gauze and secured to the skin with Allis clamps both laterally and medially. About 1 cm proximal to the metacarpophalangeal joint crease, a circumferential incision was made with more skin being preserved in the posterior aspect to use as a posterior flap. The incision was then carried down through the subcutaneous tissue. The metacarpophalangeal joint was disarticulated as the joint attachments were divided. The amputated toe was sent to Pathology. Gloves were changed. The protruding bone was trimmed with a Rongeur and filed so that the edges were smooth. The skin was apposed together and there was no significant protrusion of the bone underneath the skin. The lateral and medial dog ears were excised. The wound was irrigated with saline. The subcutaneous tissue was closed with interrupted stitches of 2-0 chronic. The skin was closed with interrupted vertical mattress stitches of 3-0 Dermalon. The patient tolerated the procedure well and was sent to the recovery room under stable conditions. On a separate table, the lymph nodes were bisected. The proximal lymph node measured 2 cm x 0.9 cm with 75% fat. A central streak of blue area was noted in the bisected lymph node, and the blue was 3/5, 75% was noted to be fat. The distal lymph node measured 2 cm x 1.1 cm. The fat was 70-75% and the blue was noted to be of 3/5. It should be noted that in the distal lymph node, the blue was noted within the fat component of the lymph node. Each bisected lymph node was sent to Pathology for histologic diagnosis. There was some fatty tissue with a count of 703 distal to the distal lymph node (Figure 9B) and this was also sent separately.

PATHOLOGY SPECIMENS: 1. Left great toe
2. Left proximal femoral SLN, 2x0.9cm, 3/5 blue, count=4663**
3. Left distal femoral SLN, 2x1.1cm, 3/5 blue, count=6601**
4. Lymphatic tissue, count = 703**

OPERATIVE COMPLICATIONS: None.
IV FLUIDS USED: Crystalloids.
DRAINS: None.
ESTIMATED BLOOD LOSS: 30-40 cc.
ASSESSMENT OF PATIENT'S CONDITION: Excellent
SURGEON:
*   A range of 1-5 cc of Lymphazurin may be given.
**   Both femoral SLNs were represented by the proximal marking and the lymphatic tissue was represented by the distal marking (Figure 9B).

Figure 10. An example of an operative report for selective sentinel lymphadenectomy for extremity melanoma.

routine histologic examination were followed expectantly with the remaining lymph nodes intact without additional lymph node dissection. Of this group of patients, 12 (2.8%) subsequently developed nodal disease within a previously mapped lymph node basin as the initial site of failure. The paraffin blocks of the SLNs from this group of patients were re-evaluated using multiserial sectioning as well as immunohistochemical staining, with monoclonal antibodies against HMB-45 and S100 melanoma-associated antigens. From these 12 patients microscopic disease was subsequently identified using more sensitive techniques. By excluding those patients who were retrospectively identified as having positive SLNs using more sensitive techniques, the long-term false-negative rate was less than 1% with median follow-up of 20 months. This data supports the contention that lymphatic mapping and selective SLN dissection accurately selects out that lymph node most likely to harbor micrometastasis.

Our study has been designed to evaluate the role of SLNs and primary melanoma high risk factors as prognostic indicators of recurrence and death in melanoma patients. Data were collected from 357 patients with invasive primary melanoma undergoing preoperative lymphoscintigraphy and intraoperative mapping of SLNs from October 21, 1993 to June 30, 1998. The overall positive SLN rate was 18% by patient count. The overall incidence of recurrence was 11% over a median follow-up period of 589 days. For negative SLN patients, 91% showed no evidence of disease (NED) and 9% had developed recurrent melanoma. For patients with positive SLNs, 77% were NED and 23% had recurrent melanoma (p=0.002). When complete lymph node dissection (CLND) was performed for patients with positive SLNs, those with positive nodes in the remaining nodal basin had a significantly shorter disease-free median survival of about 10 months (p=0.006). Of the SLN negative patients, 3% have died, 50% of them due to metastatic melanoma. For the patients with metastatic melanoma to the SLNs, 16% have died, all of them due to metastatic melanoma (p=0.016). Of the patients with a Breslow thickness less than 2.25 mm, 11% had positive SLNs, whereas 32% had positive SLNs (p<0.00005) when the Breslow thickness is 2.25 mm or greater. Angiolymphatic invasion, high mitotic index, microsatellitosis, and ulceration were also significant predictors of positive SLNs. We conclude that both micrometastasis to SLNs and some high risk factors are predictors of poor prognosis for melanoma. Micrometastasis to SLNs and subsequent non-SLNs from the CLND is associated with the worst prognosis [Leong 2000a]. We have found micrometastasis as small as a cluster of 25-50 cells may be associated with additional nodal disease in the complete lymph node dissection (unpublished data). Future adjuvant trials should be directed towards this subgroup of patients. This data supports the fact that lymphatic mapping and selective SLN dissection not only accurately select out that lymph node most likely to harbor micrometastasis, but also may be used as a tool to prognosticate the clinical outcome.

CURRENT STATUS

The selective SLN dissection in melanoma should be considered a standard approach [Reintgen 1996, Coit 1997, Emilia 1997, Houghton 1998] for staging primary malignant melanoma, provided that the surgeons, nuclear medicine physicians and pathologists are adequately trained [Morton 1999]. Because the false-negative rate is extremely low, it can be assumed that those patients with a negative SLN should have no microscopic disease in the remainder of their nodal basin. Therefore, selective SLN dissection allows about 80% of patients with melanoma to be spared a formal lymph node dissection, thus, avoiding the complications usually associated with that procedure.

Because of the relative ease of assessing the SLNs with a less invasive procedure than a formal lymphadenectomy, it is tempting to have this information, particularly with respect to the use of interferon α-2b (Schering, Kenilworth, NJ), for the adjuvant treatment of patients with stage III melanoma who are at a high risk for recurrence (defined as those patients with metastatic lymph nodes)[Kirkwood 1996]. Selective SLN dissection has been suggested as an alternative to prophylactic lymph node dissection as means of assessing regional lymph node metastatic status [Reintgen 1996].

OVERVIEW

Several advantages of SLNs in malignant melanoma [Rivers 1997] include: 1) a negative SLN biopsy will reduce the extent of surgery, cost, and morbidity for many patients with primary malignant melanoma who might otherwise be told to have an elective lymph node dissection; 2) the removal of a positive SLN followed by a prophylatic lymph node dissection will provide better local control of the disease-involved lymphatic basin; 3) a selective sentinel lymphadenectomy can be considered as staging procedure when it is positive, after which additional surgery and adjuvant treatment such as interferon α-2b may be given; 4) a negative sentinel lymphadenectomy may reassure the patient that the likelihood of metastatic disease to the regional lymph node is low. Therefore, it offers considerable psychological benefit.

Clearly, the role of SLN dissection is to provide accurate staging at the initial diagnosis of primary melanoma. In order to enhance such accuracy, it requires: 1) accurate identification and localization of SLN by preoperative lymphoscintigraphy and intraoperative mapping and dissection, and 2) meticulous histological evaluation by serial sectioning [Robert 1993, Lane 1958, Das Gupta 1977, Wang 1994] on one or a few SLNs as routine histologic techniques for routine evaluation of lymph nodes may decrease the diagnostic accuracy mainly because of sampling errors [Reintgen 1995]. Serial sectioning would be too exhaustive to be done on multiple nodes from ELND.

To achieve a high rate of accurate and successful identification of the SLNs, it is imperative that the surgeons, physicians of nuclear medicine, and pathologists work together closely as a multidisciplinary team to offer the best result to the patient.

PEARLS

- The lymph node is usually below the fascia. (e.g. clavipectoral fascia in the axilla and Scarpa's fascia in the groin.) So, a tunneling and not a flap type of incision should be developed to gain access to the fascia. The Baily right angle is a excellent instrument for dissection. The Allis clamp is routinely used to grasp the adjacent tissue surrounding the SLN to lift it from deep into the operative field. Dissection should be as close to the lymph node as possible to avoid injuries to the adjacent nerves and vessels.

- For dissection of SLN in the parotid or spinal accessory nerve area, it is important to use a nerve stimulator to guide the dissection to avoid nerve injury.

- The lymph nodes may be in any portion of the wall of the cavity as the tunnel is being dissected, especially with respect to the second or the third SLN. Therefore, the roaming counts are very important, particularly if the preoperative lymphoscintigraphy shows there are two or three SLNs. Roaming counts are important to have a panoramic search for any additional SLNs. A resection bed count alone may not find additional residual SLNs.

- If the reading is very focal with disappearance of counts with minimal motion of the probe, the lymph node is usually small. When the SLN is small, say 5 mm or so in a large basin such as axilla, it would be somewhat difficult to find it because with further dissection, the tissue is loosening, the tissue may be folding over and that lymph node may be hidden away in a sort a "blind spot" which may not be detected. Sometimes it can be frustrating that occasionally when your probe comes into contact with that lymph node there is a transient registration of an elevated count. On the other hand, when you try to go back again, it is not there. Obviously, patience is needed to find such a SLN.

- If the reading disappears after retraction, use shallower retractors. This indicates that the lymph node is in a superficial plane.

- When the first SLN has been found which is usually quite easy because at this point, tissue of dissection is limited and there is quite a bit of integrity of the tissue to help to dissect that particular SLN. By the time when the second or third SLN is to be dissected, the cavity architecture is now loose. It makes the identification by the Neoprobe of the SLN more difficult to localize it. Therefore, it takes patience and vigilance to find the second or third SLN.

- It should be noted that for the blue dye during initial encountering of it in vivo, it may appear to be 3 to 4 plus blue and during dissection the blue may decrease in intensity. On the other hand, the radioisotope count on the lymph node remains stable during the in vivo reading and ex-vivo reading.

- When the nuclear medicine physician recognizes a SLN, it could represent a cluster of a few lymph nodes.

- A collimator may be used to minimize "shine through effect" from the adjacent primary injection site being close to the SLN site. When a collimator is used, the field of detection is more focal and limited. For a more panoramic search, the collimator may be detached.

- Different sizes of the retractors should be used in order to gain access to the SLN guided by gamma probe. Once the SLN is identified by a gamma probe, an Allis clamp can be used to grasp the adjacent tissue of the lymph node without crushing it so it can be lifted up into the operative field for dissection. Alternatively a silk stitch can be used, but the author finds that an Allis clamp is more reliable and more secure than a silk stitch, especially if the lymph node is deep, for example, in the axilla.

- It is not clear whether a deep external illiac lymph node should be explored initially if identified by preoperative lymphoscintigraphy. The author's approach is that the superficial ingual lymph nodes should be harvested only if the superficial and deep iliac nodes are contiguous. If they are positive, at the time of completion lymph node dissection the patient would then undergo an illioingual lymph node dissection. On the other hand, when a separate channel leads to a deep ilian node, it will be harvested separately.

- For anatomical sites which are difficult to triangulate for marking preopreatively by the nuclear medicine physician including the lower neck, upper back, epitrochlear, popliteal and any in-transit area, it is important to do a careful mapping by the hand-held gamma probe prior to making the incision. Particularly, this is relevant in the upper back area where the lymph node could be in the supraclavicular area and yet the marking is in the upper back trapezius area. Also, in the upper arm for the epitrochlear area, the actual lymph node may be in a different location than the preoperative lymphoscintigraphic marking would indicate.

- Digital exploration should always be done prior to the completion of selective sentenel lymphadenectomy to make sure that no suspicious or enlarged lymph nodes are retained in the surgical bed as blue dye or radiocolloid may not enter a grossly metastatic lymph node.

REFERENCES

Albertini JJ, Cruse CW, Rapaport D, et al. Intraoperative radio-lympho-scintigraphy improves sentinel lymph node identification for patients with melanoma. Annals of Surgery 1996;223(2):217-24

Alex JC, Krag DN. Gamma-probe-guided localization of lymph nodes. Surgical Oncology 1993;2(3):137-44

Balch CM, Soong S, Ross MI, et al. Long-term results of a multi-institutional randomized trial comparing prognostic factors and surgical results for intermediate thickness melanomas (1.0 to 4.0mm). Annals of Surgical Oncology 2000;7(2):87-97

Balch CM, Soong S, Bartolucci A, et al. Efficacy of an elective regional lymph node dissection of 1 to 4 mm thick melanomas for patients 60 years of age and younger. Annals of Surgery 1996;224(3):255-66

Balch CM. The role of elective lymph node dissection in melanoma: rationale, results and controversies. Journal of Clinical Oncology 1988;6(1):163-72

Balch CM, Soong SJ, Murad TN, et al. A multifactorial analysis of melanoma: III. Prognostic factors in melanoma patients with lymph node metastases (stage II). Annals of Surgery 1981;193(3):377-88

Berman CG, Norman J, Cruse CW, et al. Lymphoscintigraphy in malignant melanoma. Annals of Plastic Surgery 1992;28(1):29-32

Bonenkamp JJ, Logan DR, Suemnig AA, Thompson JF. The cost of sentinel node biopsy (SNB) for melanoma. [Abstract] Melanoma Research 2001; 11(Supplement 1):S107

Bostick P, Essner R, Sarantou T, et al. Intraoperative lymphatic mapping for early-stage melanoma of the head and neck. American Journal of Surgery 1997;174(5):536-539

Callery C, Cochran AJ, Roen DJ, et al. Factors prognostic for survival in patients with malignant melanoma spread to the regional lymph nodes. Annals of Surgery 1982;196(1):69-75

Cohen MH, Ketcham AS, Felix EL. Prognostic factors in patients undergoing lymphadenectomy for malignant melanoma. Annals of Surgery 1977;186(5):635-42

Coit D, Wallack M, Balch C. Society of Surgical Oncology practice guidelines. Melanoma surgical practice guidelines. Oncology 1997;11(9):1317-23

Coldiron B. No evidence to support delay in excision of malignant melanoma. [Letter] Archives of Dermatology 2000;136(10):1269-70

Das Gupta TK. Results of treatment of 269 patients with primary cutaneous melanoma: a five-year prospective study. Annals of Surgery 1977;186:201-9

Emilia JCD, Lawrence W. Sentinel lymph node biopsy in malignant melanoma: The standard of care? Journal of Surgical Oncology 1997;65(3):153-4

Eshima D, Fauconnier T, Eshima L, et al. Radiopharmaceuticals for Lymphoscintigraphy: Including Dosimetry and Radiation Considerations. Seminars in Nuclear Medicine 2000;30(1):25-32

Fee HJ, Robinson DS, Sample WF, et al. The determination of lymph shed by colloidal gold scanning patients with malignant melanoma: a preliminary study. Surgery 1978;84(5):626-32

Gershenwald JE, Thompson W, Mansfield PF, et al. Multi-institutional melanoma lymphatic mapping experience: the prognostic value of sentinel lymph node status in 612 stage I or II melanoma patients. Journal of Clinical Oncology 1999;17(3):976-83

Glass LF, Messina JL, Cruse W, et al: The use of intraoperative radiolymphoscintigraphy for sentinel node biopsy in patients with malignant melanoma. Dermatologic Surgery 1996;22(8):715-20

Glass FL, Fenske NA, Messina JL, et al. The role of selective lymphadenectomy in the management of patients with malignant melanoma. Dermatologic Surgery 1995;21(11):979-83

Houghton A, Coit D, Bloomer W, et al. NCCN melanoma practice guidelines. National Comprehensive Cancer Network. Oncology 1998;12(7a):153-77

Joseph E, Messina J, Glass FL, et al. Radioguided surgery for the ultrastaging of the patient with melanoma. Cancer Journal 1997;3(6):341-5

Kapteijn BA, Nieweg OE, Liem I, et al. Localizing the sentinel node in cutaneous melanoma: gamma probe detection versus blue dye. Annals of Surgical Oncology 1997;4(2):156-60

Karakousis CP. Surgical Treatment of Malignant Melanoma. In: Leong SPL, editor. Surgical Clinics of North America: Cutaneous Malignant Melanoma. Philadelphia: WB Saunders, 1996a;76(6):1299-312

Karakousis CP, Velez AF, Spellman JE, Jr., et al. The technique of sentinel node biopsy. European Journal of Surgical Oncology 1996b;22(3):271-5

Kirkwood JM, Strawderman MH, Ernstoff MS. Interferon alpha-2b adjuvant therapy of high-risk resected cutaneous melanoma: the Eastern Cooperative Oncology Group Trial EST 1684. Journal of Clinical Oncology 1996;14(1):7-17

Kowalsky RJ, Perry JR. Radiopharmaceuticals in Nuclear Medicine Practice. Los Altos: Appleton and Lange; 1987.

Krag DN, Meijer SJ, Weaver DL, et al. Minimal-access surgery for staging of malignant melanoma. Archives of Surgery 1995;130(6):654-8

Krouse RS, Schwarz RE. Blue dye for sentinel lymph node mapping: not too sensitive, but too hypersensitive? [Letter]. Annals of Surgical Oncology. In press 2000.

Lamki LM, Logic JR. Defining lymphatic drainage patterns with cutaneous lymphoscintigraphy. In: Balch CM, Hougton AN, Milton GW, et al, editors. Cutaneous Melanoma. 2nd ed. Philadelphia: J.B. Lippincott; 1992. p 367-75.

Lane N, Lattes R, Malm J. Clinicopathological correlation in a series of 117 malignant melanomas of the skin of adults. Cancer 1958;11:1025-43

Leong SPL, Acthem T, Miller J, et al. Clinical Significance of Melanoma Micrometastasis to Sentinel Lymph Nodes and Other High Risk Factors. [Abstract] Proceedings of the American Society of Clinical Oncology; New Orleans, LA. 2000a.

Leong SPL, Donegan E, Heffernon W, et al. Adverse reactions to isosulfan blue during selective sentinel lymph node dissection in melanoma. Annals of Surgical Oncology 2000b;7:361-366

Leong SPL. Blue dye for sentinel lymph node mapping: not too sensitive, but too hypersensitive? [Letter, Reply] Annals of Surgical Oncology. In press 2000c.

Leong SPL, Nguyen L, Morita E, et al. Superiority of Radiocolloid over Isosulfan Blue Dye in the Detection of Melanoma Sentinel Lymph Nodes. [Abstract] 2nd International Sentinel Node Congress; Santa Monica, CA. December, 2000d

Leong SPL. No evidence to support delay in excision of malignant melanoma. [Letter, Reply] Archives of Dermatology 2000e; 136(10):1269-70

Leong SPL, Habib FA, Achtem TA, et al. Discordancy between clinical predictions versus lymphoscintigraphic and intraoperative mapping of sentinel lymph node drainage of primary melanoma. Archives of Dermatology 1999a;135(12):1472-6

Leong SPL, Steinmetz I, Habib FA, et al. Optimal selective sentinel lymph node dissection in primary malignant melanoma. Archives of Surgery 1997;132(6):666-73

Lingam MK, Mackie RM, McKay AJ. Intraoperative identification of sentinel lymph node in patients with malignant melanoma. British Journal of Cancer 1997;75(10):1505-8

McNeer G, Das Gupta TK. Prognosis in malignant melanoma. Surgery 1964;56:512-8

Meyer CM, Lecklitner ML, Logic JR, et al. Technetium-99m sulfur-colloid cutaneous lymphoscintigraphy in the management of truncal melanoma. Radiology 1979;131(1):205-9

Morton DL, Chan AD. Current status of intraoperative lymphatic mapping and sentinel lymphadenectomy for melanoma: is it standard of care? Journal of the American College of Surgeons 1999;189(2):214-23

Morton DL, Wen DR, Cochran AJ. Management of early stage melanoma by intraoperative lymphatic mapping and selective lymphadenectomy. In: Coit DG, editor. Surgical Oncology Clinics of North America: Lymph Node Dissection in Malignant Melanoma. Philadelphia: WB Saunders, 1992a;1(2):247-59

Morton DL, Wen DR, Wong JH, et al. Technical details of intraoperative lymphatic mapping for early stage melanoma. Archives of Surgery 1992b;127(4):392-9

Pijpers R, Borgstein PJ, Meijer S, et al. Sentinel node biopsy in melanoma patients: dynamic lymphoscintigraphy followed by intraoperative gamma probe and vital dye guidance. World Journal of Surgery 1997;21(8):788-92, discussion 793

Pijpers R, Collet GJ, Meijer S, et al. The impact of dynamic lymphoscintigraphy and gamma probe guidance on sentinel node biopsy in melanoma. European Journal of Nuclear Medicine 1995;22(11):1238-41

Reintgen DS. Changing standards of surgical care for melanoma patients. Annals of Surgical Oncology 1996;3:327-8

Reintgen D, Albertini J, Berman, et al. Accurate nodal staging of malignant melanoma. Cancer Control Journal of Moffitt Cancer Center 1995;2:405-14

Reintgen DS, Cruse CW, Wells K. The orderly progression of melanoma nodal metastases. Annals of Surgery 1994;220(6):759-67

Rivers JK, Roof MI. Sentinel lymph-node biopsy in melanoma: is less surgery better? Lancet 1997;350(9088):1336-7

Robert M, Wen D, Cochran A. Pathological evaluation of the regional lymph nodes in malignant melanoma. Seminars in Diagnostic Pathology 1993;10(1):102-15

Roses DF, Provet JA, Harris MN, et al. Prognosis of patients with pathologic stage II cutaneous malignant melanoma. Annals of Surgery 1985;201(1):103-7

Ross MI, Reintgen DS, Balch C. Selective lymphadenectomy: Emerging role for lymphatic mapping and sentinel node biopsy in the management of early stage melanoma. Seminars in Surgical Oncology 1993;9(3):219-23

Sim FH, Taylor WF, Ivins JC, et al. A prospective randomized study of the efficacy of routine elective lymphadenectomy in management of malignant melanoma: preliminary results. Cancer 1978;41(3):948-56

Sullivan DC, Croker BP, Harris CC, et al. Lymphoscintigraphy in malignant melanoma: 99mTc antimony sulfur colloid. American Journal of Roentgenology 1981;137(4):847-51

Thompson JF, McCarthy WH, Bosch CM, et al. Sentinel lymph node status as an indicator of the presence of metastatic melanoma in regional lymph nodes. Melanoma Research 1995;5(4):255-60

Thompson J, McCarthy W, Robinson E. Sentinel lymph node biopsy in 102 patients with clinical stage I melanoma undergoing elective lymph node dissection, 47th Cancer symposium Society of Surgical Oncology. Houston, Texas, 1994.

Uren DF, Howman-Giles RB, Shaw HM, et al. Lymphoscintigraphy in high risk melanoma of the trunk: Predicting draining node groups, defining lymphatic channels and locating the sentinel node. Journal of Nuclear Medicine 1993;34(9):1435-40

Van der Veen H, Hoekstra O, Paul M, et al. Gamma probe-guided sentinel node biopsy to select patients with melanoma for lymphadenectomy. British Journal of Surgery 1994;81(12):1769-70

Veronesi U, Adamus J, Bandiera DC. Inefficacy of immediate node dissection in stage I melanoma of the limbs. New England Journal of Medicine 1977;297(12):627-30

Wanebo HJ, Harpole D, Teates CD. Radionuclide lymphoscintigraphy with technetium 99m antimony sulfide colloid to identify lymphatic drainage of cutaneous melanoma at abiguous sites in the head and neck and trunk. Cancer 1985;55(6):1403-13

Wang X, Heller R, VanVoorheis N, et al. Detection of submicroscopic lymph node metastases with polymerase chain reaction in patients with malignant melanoma. Annals of Surgery 1994;220(6):768-74

Wells KE, Rapaport DP, Cruse CW, et al. Sentinel lymph node biopsy in melanoma of the head and neck. Plastic and Reconstructive Surgery 1997;100(3):591-4

White DC, Schuler FR, Pruitt SK, et al. Timing of sentinel lymph node mapping after lymphoscintigraphy. Surgery 1999;126(2):156-61

4 SELECTIVE SENTINEL LYMPH NODE MAPPING AND DISSECTION FOR BREAST CANCER

Stanley P. L. Leong, MD

RATIONALE FOR SELECTIVE SENTINEL LYMPHADENECTOMY FOR BREAST CANCER

In 1994, Giuliano [1994] and coworkers published the initial report of the use of a vital blue dye for the purpose of intraoperative lymphatic mapping and sentinel node dissection for invasive breast cancer following the model system of melanoma [Morton 1997]. Since that initial report, a number of studies have confirmed the concept of sentinel lymph node (SLN) in breast cancer [Giuliano 1999b]. In other words, when breast cancer metastasizes to regional lymph nodes, it most frequently goes to the SLN. If the SLN is free from micrometastasis by both hematoxylin and eosin and immunohistochemical staining, the probability of non-sentinel node detection of tumor cells is <0.1%. The true false-negative rate of this technique using multiple sections and immunohistochemical staining to detect micrometastasis is 0.97% (1/103). Therefore, it is concluded that the SLN is indeed the most probable lymph node to harbor metastatic breast carcinoma [Turner 1997]. The concept of SLN has been currently applied to breast cancer as shown in Table 1.

Table 1. Summary of Selective Sentinel Lymphadectomy in Breast Cancer from the Literature *

Study	# of Pts	Mapping Technique	Sensitivity %	Diagnostic Accuracy %	False No.	Negative %
Giuliano, et al. [1994]	114	B**	88	95.6	5	6.5
Krag, et al. [1993]	18	Tc***	100	100	0	0
Veronesi, et al. [1997]	160	Tc	95.3	97.5	4	5.1
Pijpers, et al. [1997]	34	Tc	100	100	0	0
Neiweg, et al. [1996]	22	B	100	100	0	0
Schneebaum, et al. [1996]	13	B/Tc	75	92.3	1	10
Guenther, et al. [1997]	103	B	90.3	97.1	3	4.2
Giuliano, et al. [1997b]	100	B	100	100	0	0
Borgstein, et al. [1998]	104	Tc	97.8	99	1	1.7
Barnwell, et al. [1998]	38	B/Tc	100	100	0	0
O'Hea, et al. [1998]	55	B/Tc	86.9	94.5	3	9.4
Cox, et al. [1998]	167	B/Tc	98.1	99.4	1	0.9

* Adapted from Leong SPL, et al. [Leong 2000a]
**B—Blue Dye (isosulfan blue) ***Tc—Technetium labeled colloid

The standard treatment for patients with primary invasive breast cancer with clinically negative nodes is adequate excision of the primary tumor either through a lumpectomy or a mastectomy and a lymph node dissection including at least levels I and II [Bland 1996]. Therefore, if SLNs can be reliably harvested for assessment of the nodal basin, the axillary lymph node dissection may potentially be avoided.

EVOLVING TECHNIQUES IN BREAST CANCER SLN MAPPING

Although Giuliano et al. showed an excellent harvesting rate of 96% using the blue dye technique [Giuliano 1999b], most other studies have reported an overall rate of about 80% [Giuliano 1999b]. With the use of radiotracer and preoperative lymphoscintigraphy, the harvesting rate of the SLN can be increased to almost 95% [Giuliano 1999b]. However, initial studies using peritumoral injection of radiotracer were met with technical problems of not identifying the SLN preoperatively or intraoperatively on a consistent basis because of the significant "shine through effect" from the peritumoral injection site especially in the upper outer quadrant. It then became a challenge to improve the injection site in order to maximize the location of the SLN and minimize the "shine through effect". Currently, in published literature, there is no standardization among investigators of the radiotracers with respect to such variations as particle size, time of injection, volume of injection, technique of preoperative lymphoscintigraphy, and choice of blue dye versus radiotracer.

Veronesi et al. [1997] was the first to report such a high success rate of 98% in the localization of the SLN by preoperative lymphoscintigraphy and surgical harvesting of the SLN using subcutaneous injection. With respect to their definition of subcutaneous injection, it is unclear as to whether it is indeed subcutaneous or rather intradermal. Borgstein first used intradermal injection of blue dye into the subareolar area of the breast regardless of the tumor location [Borgstein 1997]. Although the success rate was reliable and high, Guiliano [1997] commented that there was a relatively permanent tattooing effect of the blue dye. Despite this concern, Borgstein's study was the first to propose the concept of "hitchhiking" or bypassing the breast parenchymal lymphatic system by exploiting the intradermal route. A review of the lymphatic system of the breast by Haagensen and others [Haagensen 1972, Grant 1959, Turner-Warwick 1953] showed a well-structured system which was very carefully defined by studies based on postmortem injection of colloid gold particles [Sappey 1874, Rouviere 1932], and by information collected from axillary draining lymph nodes based on mastectomy specimens [Haagensen 1972]. Indeed, the parenchymal lymphatic system is connected through a lymphatic network to the cutaneous and periareolar lymphatic channels leading to the corresponding SLN. Therefore, if the entire pathway is connected, then any point of injection in the lymphatic network such as intradermal injection over the skin of the breast lesion, or periareolar injection would probably drain to the same SLN as if injected peritumorally. Since the lymphatic channels are much richer at the cutaneous level than the peritumoral site, it is much easier to "light up" the SLN by lymphoscintigraphy using the intradermal or periareolar injections. Thus, Linehan et al. showed [Linehan 1999] that the dermal and parenchymal lymphatics of the breast drain to the same SLN in most patients. Also, Klimberg et al. showed that subareolar injection of technetium is as accurate as peritumoral injection of blue dye [Klimberg 1999]. The subareolar approach has been further confirmed by Kern and Rosenberg [Kern 2000] to be reliable. Furthermore, Roumen used both peritumoral and intradermal radiotracer injections [Roumen 1999], either in the skin overlying the tumor or periareolerly in the quadrant of the tumor, with dynamic and static images to match or mismatch the hot spots visualized by both techniques. Roumen showed that the skin and peritumorally injection go to the same axillary sentinel node with few exceptions [Roumen 1999].

Both peritumoral and intradermal injections will result in an excellent match of the axillary SLN but the internal mammary lymph nodes are not visualized with intradermal injections. On the other hand, the periareolar area may identify an internal mammary chain [Vendrell-Torne 1972]. From our experience with melanoma in the upper anterior trunk area, using intradermal injections, the internal mammary node has not been appreciated. In our own expereince with breast cancer patients, no internal mammary nodes were seen in 50 out of 50 patients from an intradermal injection. On the other hand, of the 35 breast cancer patients with peritumoral injections, 6 patients showed the presence of internal mammary lymph nodes (17%). To date, our policy is not to explore the internal mammary nodes, although the lymphatic mapping technique for internal mammary nodes has been recently described [Harlow 1999]. The issue of identifying internal mammary nodes remains controversial and only prospective studies will address the significance of the internal mammary lymph nodes [Harlow 1999]. In general, if the axillary lymph node basin is negative, the internal mammary nodes are usually negative. Therefore, if the axillary SLN is negative, the internal mammary nodes may be assumed to be negative.

Based on the classic description of the breast lymphatic system [Haagensen 1972] and recent studies by Linehan [1999], Klimberg [1999], Roumen [1999], and Kern [2000] concordancy between peritumoral and dermal/periareolar lymphatic drainage to the same SLN is probably the rule.

In our experience at UCSF Medical Center at Mount Zion with a subgroup of 35 patients with peritumoral injection, the SLN was identified by lymphoscintigraphy within 10 minutes. But in three patients, the SLN was not seen from 3 to 24 hours. In about 50 patients when intradermal injection is given, the SLN was seen within 10 minutes and many times seen almost immediately after the injection. The rate of identifying SLN by intradermal injection is much higher than by peritumoral injection (98.5% versus 75%) [Leong manuscript in preparation]. Further, the concordancy rate between intradermal and peritumoral injection was 100% in 9 patients who had peritumoral injection on the day before surgery and intradermal injection the next day. Recent multicenter study shows that intradermal injection of radioactive colloid significantly improves the SLN identification rate [McMasters 2001].

We have observed that after blue dye injection into the peritumoral areas that the blue comes to the surface above the tumor site and then goes to the axillary SLNs (Figure 1) attesting to the fact that lymphatic channels in the breast maybe connected between the parenchymal tissue and the overlying skin.

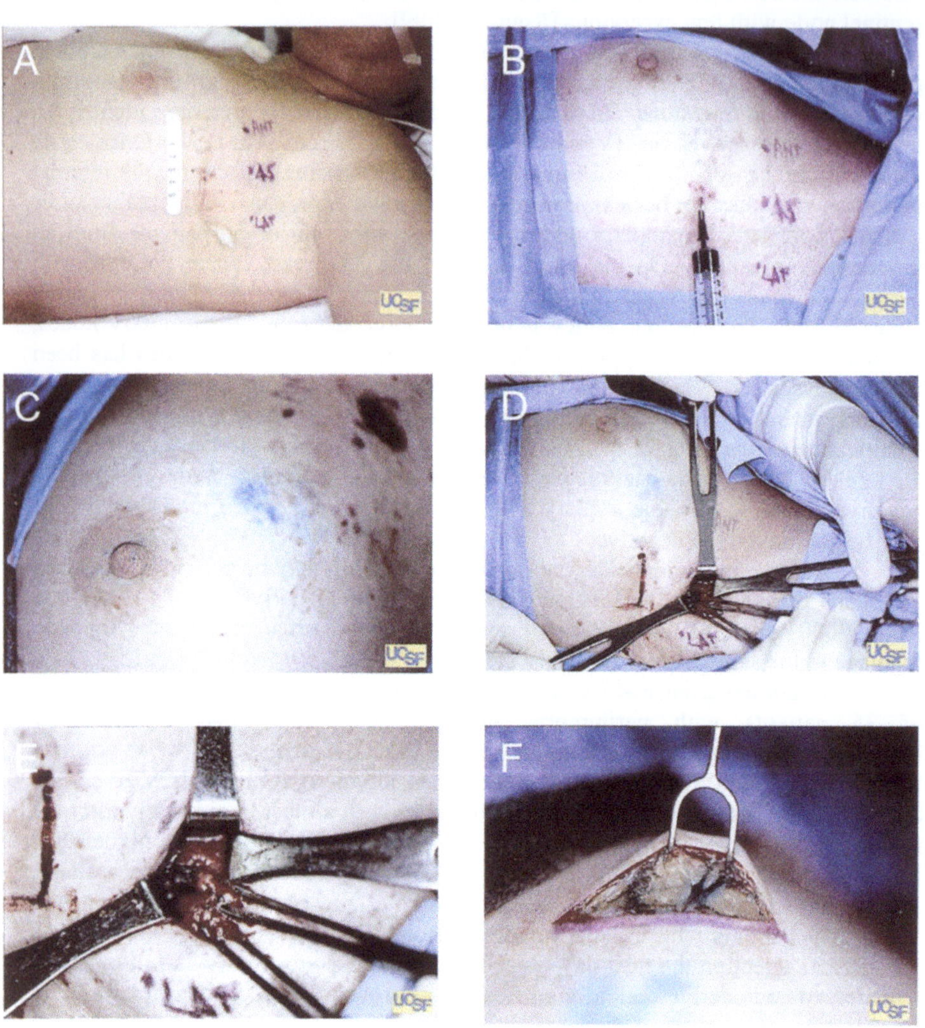

Figure 1. Intraoperative peritumoral injection of blue dye results in the appearance of the blue dye to the skin and periareolar area and subsequently to the SLN. (See Figure 2 for detailed operative report.)

SELECTIVE SENTINEL LYMPH NODE MAPPING FOR BREAST CANCER: HOW WE DO IT

I. Preoperative Lymphoscintigraphy

The use of the gamma camera to localize the SLN is important although Krag states that imaging is not necessary [Krag 1998]. At UCSF Medical Center at Mount Zion, we have developed a close working relationship between the nuclear medicine physician and the surgical staff. The imaging information is communicated to the surgeon prior to selective SLN dissection. This practice gives the surgeon a greater confidence in localizing the lymph node. In-transit nodes for consideration are noted. Although Krag has defined nodes with ease using the gamma probe alone, we consider preoperative imaging with precise marking of the patient's skin of the position of the SLN shortens the time of search and facilitates the harvesting of the SLN.

Preparation of Tc99m Sulfur Colloid

The sulfur colloid is made by a hydrogen sulfide technique [Kowalsky 1987], which makes the particles much smaller than the standard thiosulfate method [Kowalsky 1987]. The radiocolloid is filtered through a 22-μm filter to remove any large particles.

Injection of sulfur colloid

For peritumoral injections, the needle tip of the wire localization is palpated near the tumor bed or the biopsy site and injected at four quadrants (1-2cc per quadrant) around the site. In order to reduce the large area of radioactivity, we inject a small volume at the site followed by 1 to 1.5 cc of saline. This tends to reduce the area of the "shine through effect". The "shine through" phenomenon can be minimized by the use of shielding techniques, movement of the breast away from the axilla, and use of different collimators such as the medium energy collimator and pinhole collimator. The medium energy collimator eliminates the artifact of septal penetration, which can cause linear artifacts that obscure the axilla and other basins. The pinhole collimator can be used to define areas closely, and direct the surgeon toward a SLN close to the injection site. When the typical lymphoscintigram shows a large node, the pinhole collimator often defines a cluster of nodes. This information alerts the surgeon to seek the additional nodes in the cluster. Alternatively, intradermal injection of the skin overlying the tumor may be performed. The injection of the skin at a single site with a dose of 0.1 to 0.3cc reduces the problem of the "shine through effect".

Identification of Lymphatic Basins

Preoperative lymphoscintigraphic identification of the axillary SLN is critical for subsequent operative harvesting of the SLN. When we combined the UCSF and University of Hawaii database of 204 breast cancer patients, the ability to harvest the SLN was significantly increased from 40.9% to 95.6 % (p<0.0005) when the SLN was identified by preoperative lymphoscintigraphy [Leong 2000a].

II. Intraoperative Mapping Technique

Lymphazurin Injection

Once the axillary SLN is identified preoperatively by lymphoscintigraphy, it may be harvested by using a hand-held gamma probe such as Neoprobe 2000 (Neoprobe Corporation, Dublin, OH). Immediately prior to breast surgery, peritumoral injection using 5cc of Lymphazurin (Hirsh Industries, Inc., Richmond Virginia) may be performed and followed by external massage of the injected area of the breast according to the method of Giuliano [1994].

Types of Anesthesia

General anesthesia has been used most frequently over 90% of the time.

Intraoperative Mapping

Usually, a transverse incision of 2-3 cm is made in the mid axilla according to the preoperative marking by the nuclear medicine physician based on the findings of preoperative lymphoscintigraphy. A tunnel type of dissection is performed rather than raising the skin flap as in a formal axillary lymph node dissection. Once the tunnel is created and the clavipectoral fascia is incised the gamma probe is inserted to localize the "hot" SLN. Its elevated ex vivo count and a low resection bed count indicates that the SLN has been harvested. Simultaneously, blue lymphatics may be traced to a blue lymph node for search of a SLN. A second SLN may be present if the resection bed count is still high [Leong 1997] (See Chapter 3).

Identification of SLNs

After SLNs are harvested, the wound is closed in a similar way as described in Chapter 3 without placement of a drain. It is important for the surgeon to label the SLN versus non-SLN accurately by using a table dissection method as described in Chapter 3 for subsequent pathologic studies.

III. Instruments

See Chapter 3.

IV. Case Illustration

A 47 year old Caucasian female presented with an abnormal mammogram taken in April 1999 of left upper outer breast. A stereotactic core biopsy two weeks prior to surgery revealed infiltrating ductal carcinoma. Chest x-ray and blood tests were unremarkable. The patient underwent a preoperative ultrasound-guided needle localization followed by lymphoscintigraphy. A SLN in the left axilla was localized by lymphoscintigraphy following intradermal injection of radiocolloid. No activity was noted in the internal mammary or supraclavicular lymph node chains. Intraoperative lymphatic mapping consisting of peritumoral injection of Isosulfan blue dye (4 cc) resulted in the migration of blue dye towards the skin and into the periareolar area within the first 10 minutes (Figure 1). Using a hand-held gamma probe as a guide, 2 SLNs were successfully harvested. One of the sentinel nodes (hot and blue) was later found to harbor micrometastasis. The other SLN (blue only) was negative. Three adjacent non-sentinel nodes were found within the specimen. A sample operative report is included (Figure 2).

Patient Name: Patient from Figure 1   MRN: #

PREOPERATIVE DIAGNOSIS: Left breast carcinoma, upper outer quadrant.

POSTOPERATIVE DIAGNOSIS: Left breast carcinoma, upper outer quadrant.

OPERATION: 1. Left axillary selective sentinel lymph node dissection and intraoperative
                    lymphatic mapping procedure.
                    2. Left breast lumpectomy.

ANESTHESIA: General endotracheal anesthesia.

CLINICAL INDICATIONS: This is a 47-year-old Caucasian female with a history of abnormal mammogram of the left upper outer breast. A core biopsy revealed infiltrating ductal carcinoma. She has no evidence of metastatic disease. Therefore, the patient was admitted for the procedures as listed above.

WOUND PREPARATION: All surgical sites were painted with Betadine and draped in the usual sterile fashion.

DESCRIPTION OF OPERATION: The patient was admitted to Nuclear Medicine for preoperative lymphoscintigraphy following needle localization in the Radiology Department. A total of 850 microcuries of Tc99 sulfur colloid were injected intradermally over the needle localized site in the left upper outer breast. Drainage was noted to a single sentinel lymph node in the left axilla. Informed consent was signed and the patient was brought to the Operating Room and placed in the supine position. I was present during the entire procedure. After satisfactory general endotracheal anesthesia was obtained, preoperative readings were taken with the Neoprobe 2000 and recorded on the data sheet. At 14:32, 4 cc of Lymphazurin were injected intratumorally. Minutes later, blue lymphatics were noted on the surface of the skin and in the periareolar area (Figure 1).

Attention was first directed to the left axilla. At 14:40, a 3 cm transverse incision was made 1.0 cm above the 45 degree marking in the left breast. At 14:45, blue lymphatics were noted 1.5 cm deep. At 14:52, a blue sentinel lymph node (3/5 blue) was secured in the mid-axilla after the clavipectoral fascia was incised with an in vivo reading of 3468. Blunt and sharp dissection was performed with hemoclips as ligatures. Hemostasis was controlled by electrocoagulation. Two blue lymphatics were noted entering this SLN. During dissection, the blue dye started to fade. The specimen of ex vivo count 2786 was removed at 15:20. The specimen contained at least two SLN's, one with fading blue dye and another persistent blue node. The resection bed was 9. Roaming counts showed increased radioactivity towards the injection site and this was considered to be shine effect. Digital exploration showed no residual suspicious or enlarged lymph nodes in the surgical bed. No further exploration was pursued. The wound was irrigated with saline. The deep subcutaneous layer was closed with interrupted stitches of 3-0 Dexon. The superficial subcutaneous layer was closed with interrupted stitches of 3-0 Dexon. The skin was closed with running subcuticular stitches of 4-0 Dexon. The wound was cleaned with saline and dried. Steri-strips were applied and a 2 x 2 gauze was placed and reinforced with a Tegaderm.

Gloves and instruments were changed. Attention was directed to the left breast biopsy site. At 16:22, a circumferential incision was made from the 1:30 o'clock to the 2:30 o'clock position at about 7 cm from the nipple. The wire was secured and the incision was followed along the wire for a distance of about 3 cm. The wire tip was secured with an Allis clamp and excision was accomplished with a 2 cm radius margin. Hemostasis was controlled by electrocoagulation. Orientation sutures were placed: a long stitch was positioned at the superior aspect, 12 o'clock, and the short stitch was positioned at the medial aspect, 9 o'clock. The blue stitch was placed at the deep margin. The excised specimen measured 4.5 cm x 6.5 cm x 4 cm. Two hemoclips were placed at the bed of the lumpectomy site for subsequent radiation boost. Gloves were changed. The wound was irrigated with saline. The superficial subcutaneous layer was closed with interrupted stitches of 3-0 Dexon. The skin was closed with running subcuticular stitches of 4-0 Dexon. The wound was cleaned with saline and dried. Steri-strips were applied and a 4 x 4 gauze was placed and reinforced with a Tegaderm. The patient tolerated the procedure well. The patient was extubated and sent to the Recovery Room under stable conditions.

On a separate table, the lymph node specimen was further dissected. Size, fat content and counts were recorded on the data base sheet. Although the first SLN was 3 to 4+ blue earlier in the surgery, the node was at most 1+ blue after dissection.

SPECIMENS TO PATHOLOGY:

1. Left axilla, SLN #1, bisected in one cassette, count = 3703, 1+ blue (both hot and blue).
2. Left axilla, non-SLN #1, bisected in one cassette, count = 5.*
3. Left axilla, non-SLN #2, bisected in one cassette, count = 7.*
4. Left axilla, non-SLN #3, bisected in one cassette, count = 8.*
5. Left axilla, SLN #2, bisected in one cassette, count = 11, 3+ blue (blue only).

6. Left breast lumpectomy specimen.
OPERATIVE COMPLICATIONS: None.   IV FLUIDS USED: Crystalloids.
DRAINS: None.   ESTIMATED BLOOD LOSS: 30 cc.
ASSESSMENT OF PATIENT'S CONDITION: Excellent.

Figure 2. An example of an operative report for intraoperative lymphatic mapping, selective axillary sentinel lymph node dissection and lumpectomy. Invasive tumor of 3cm in greatest dimension was found with clear margins. All the lymph nodes were negative except for SLN #1, which harbored a single 0.1cm microscopic focus of metastatic breast carcinoma. *These 3 non-sentinel lymph nodes were found within the SLN specimen during the table dissection.

Therefore, we feel that it is appropriate to simplify the technique by using intradermal injections. Intradermal injections overlying the tumor or periareolarly in the quadrant of the tumor may fascilitate the standardization of preoperative lymphoscintigraphy and subsequent intraoperative mapping and harvesting of the axillary SLNs.

COMPLICATIONS

Adverse reactions to blue dye are estimated to be about 1% as reported for melanoma patients [Leong 2000b]. Recently, adverse reaction to blue dye have also been reported in breast cancer SLN procedure at about 1.1% [Albo 2001]. A national survey has been conducted by the author and the results will be published [Leong manuscript in preparation]. Adverse reactions were encountered in both melanoma and breast cancer cases. The surgical and anesthesia complications are consistent to the procedure performed. Statistics are being collected in a prospective fashion as to nerve injury, wound infection, seroma, lymphadema and so forth.

CLINICAL OUTCOME

The clinical significance of the status of SLNs has yet to be determined based on follow-up of patients for regional and systemic recurrences.

CURRENT STATUS

The impact of axillary lymph node dissection on survival is controversial. Several studies show that there is no significant impact of axillary lymph node dissection on survival [Fisher 1985, CRCWP 1980, Cythgre 1982, McArdle 1986, Fisher 1989, Rutquist 1993]. On the other hand, other studies showed that the effect of local regional control by axillary lymph node dissection could be translated to overall survival [Hayward 1981, Langlands 1980, Cabanes 1992, White 1996, Overgaard 1997, Ragaz 1997, Orr 1999]. As axillary lymph node dissection is associated with significant morbidity, less invasive procedures have been attempted to diagnose axillary metastases. Should metastasis develop in the axilla, delayed lymph node dissection may be equally effective as immediate lymph node dissection on the overall survival for women with breast cancer.

To settle the controversies surrounding axillary lymph node dissection, a prospective randomized study has been devised and is being sponsored by The National Cancer Institute and the American College of Surgeons Oncology Group entitled "A Randomized Trial of Axillary Node Dissection in Women with Clinical T1-2 NO MO Breast Cancer Who Have a Positive SLN" (http://www.acosog.org). This randomized study has been designed to address the issue of whether or not an axillary lymph node dissection is necessary. Certainly, there would be no significant benefit of axillary lymph node dissection for patients with a negative axilla. Therefore, the patients with primary breast cancer are randomized only when a SLN is positive for micrometastisis for either an axillary lymph node dissection or no axillary node dissection to be followed by appropriate radiation and systemic therapy. If the outcome of the study shows that there is no difference in the two arms then the treatment with less morbidity and fewer complications, presumably selective SLN dissection would be the procedure of choice. Using the prospective and randomization approach the impact of axillary lymph node dissection of survival can be assessed in a prospective fashion. It is possible that after the removal of a positive SLN, no further surgery is needed for women with regional lymph node metastasis from early breast cancer. A slightly different randomized clinical trial: "A Randomized, Phase III Clinical Trial to Compare Sentinel Node Resection to Conventional Axillary Dissection in Clinically Node-Negative Breast Cancer Patients" has been launched by The National Surgical Adjuvant Breast and Bowel Project [Krag 1999]. In order to make these clinical studies successful it is required that a high standard of accuracy must be achieved by the multidisciplinary approach between the surgeons, nuclear medicine physicians, and pathologists. Indeed, a surgeon has to be qualified by performing 30 SLN dissections to be followed by a complete lymph node dissection so as to establish the false negative rate of the surgeon in him or herself to be less than 10% [Giuliano 1999a, Cox 1999].

GUIDELINES FROM THE AMERICAN SOCIETY OF BREAST SURGEONS [American Society of Breast Surgeons 2000]

Recently the American Society of Breast Surgeons published "Revised Consensus Statement on Guidelines for Performance of Sentinel Lymphadenectomy for Breast Cancer" with points which are included below:

1. Patients with palpable, suspicious, metastatic axillary lymph nodes should not be considered for sentinel lymphadenectomy (SL). In addition, SL may be unreliable for patients with multifocal malignancies, for those patients with a history of previous chemotherapy or radiation therapy for breast cancer, and for patients with histories of either extensive prior breast or axillary surgery. SL in this setting should be performed only as part of a research protocol.

2. Axillary treatment for patients with metastatic disease found in SLNs remains controversial. Until further multi-center trial results are available a staging Level I and II lymph node dissection is recommended outside of the clinical trial setting.

3. The credentialing and privileging of SL, as with any surgical procedure, are by the policies and processes of each local hospital. Each hospital will define its own criteria for accepting the findings of SL in lieu of axillary dissection and it is encouraged that this is done in partnership with an experienced staff breast surgeon. The Society recognizes the controversy regarding the level of experience sufficient for accepting the results of SL as the staging procedure of choice in the clinical setting where the results are used to determine indications for systemic therapy. Information from two national registries qualifying the community experience was presented at the year 2000 annual meeting of the American Society of Breast Surgeons. Findings from these registries indicated that an approximate 10 case experience is necessary for a $\geq 85\%$ success in identifying an axillary SLN. More importantly, data from these two databases indicates that an individual surgical experience of at least 20 cases of SL, where both SL and axillary dissection are performed, is necessary to minimize the risk of false-negative results. The false-negative rate (i.e., the ratio of the number of false-negative biopsies to the number of patients with positive lymph nodes) is the most important factor regarding accurate SLN staging. Past experience suggests an acceptable average false-negative rate in the range of 5%.

4. The impact on a surgeon's experience by proctored cases, and formal training in accredited continuing medical education courses is thought to reduce the personal case experience necessary to achieve optimal results, but is yet to be quantified.

5. After abandoning axillary dissection in favor of SL, surgeons should continue to report their axillary recurrence rate. This rate should be less than 5%. Surgeons are encouraged to report their experience by contributing to national registries and enrolling patients in clinical trials.

OVERVIEW

Selective sentinel lymphadenectomy represents a true multidisciplinary team approach to the management of the patient with invasive breast cancer. To achieve a high rate of accurate and successful identification of the SLNs, it is imperative that the surgeons, nuclear medicine physicians and pathologists work together closely as a multidisciplinary team to offer the best result to the patient. There is a general consensus that this is currently a procedure that should be performed under an internal review board protocol with approximately 20-30 cases being performed followed by a completion axillary node dissection. An analysis of the results being performed before proceeding on to SLN dissection alone is imperative to determine that sufficient quality control is in place in all aspects of the multidisciplinary approach. Standardization of techniques in lymphoscintigraphy, intraoperative lymphatic mapping and pathologic evaluation of SLNs is being developed. The clinical significance of the breast SLN still remains to be evaluated based on follow up of breast cancer patients undergoing selective SLN dissection and on patients being enrolled in clinical trials.

PEARLS

Valuable practical tips of selective sentinel lymphadenectomy for breast cancer from several experts are listed on the following page*. Some of the pearls listed in the author's chapter on melanoma (Chapter 3) regarding axillary selective SLN dissection may also apply in breast selective sentinel lymphadenectomy.

- Patients will experience almost immediate excretion of blue dye in the urine, creating a blue or blue-green color to the urine. Patients will invariably pass blue stool at some point following the lymphatic mapping procedure. It is important to inform patients of these two events to allay any fear they may experience.

- Blue dye allergic reactions do occur; watch the injection site for wheal reactions, and monitor the pulse and blood pressure during the procedure.

- Do not mix isosulfan blue dye, Tc99m-labelled sulfur colloid, or local anesthetics in the same syringe for combined injection; a precipitate will form, and neither dye nor colloid will migrate, leading to mapping failure.

- Giuliano's pearls: Inject 5 cc of isosulfan blue dye intra-parenchymally along the axillary side of the tumor or biopsy site. Apply 5 minutes of continuous, firm manual compression to the breast over the injection site, in a gentle rotating motion. Make the incision 1 cm below the axillary hairline. Proceed to the depth of the clavi-pectoral fascia, at which point proceed with caution to look for a blue channel leading to the SLN.

- For using the blue dye technique of Giuliano, usually, the blue lymph node is in the junction between the tail end of the breast and the lower level of the axilla. Usually it is about two centimeters or within that short distance underneath the skin below the subcutaneous tissue and below the layer of the superficial fascia, there will be a blue lymphatic running longitudinally towards the lower aspect of level I into a lymph node. The lymphatic channel may not be obvious and not present proximal to the lymph node and therefore if dissection is made at this level, the blue lymphatics may not be seen. To dissect further proximally and deeper either towards the latisia dorsi or towards the medial chest wall will not find the SLN. Therefore, when such deep levels are reached, it is important to regroup the situation again and think about the fact that the incision may be too high above the level of the blue lymphatics, it can be traced back to find that blue lymphatics and therefore to secure the blue lymph node.

- Schedule ample time. Perform the procedure in a calm environment. Operate in a bloodless field; use electrocautery. Have good retraction and good help. Proceed with caution; clip lymphatic channels. Do not cut a blue channel.

- Remember the inverse square law. As the gamma probe approaches the "hot" SLN, the count increases proportional to the square of the radius.

- "Shine through" occurs and can be problematic; remember where the "light bulbs" are and "keep your eye on the ball." Keep in mind where the radioactivity was injected or where it may have traveled and its relation to direction of the line of sight of the probe.

- Cox's pearls: Approximately 94% of all SLNs in breast cancer are found within a 5-cm circle; the center point is marked by the inferior border of the hairline in the axilla and a line drawn through the center of the hairbearing area, along the axis of the axilla. This point is situated where the lateral branch of the third intercostal nerve crosses the central axillary vein, beneath the clavi-pectoral fascia.

- Reintgen's pearl: Identification of the SLN is certain when there is an area of clearly diminished counts between the injection site and the "hot spot" in the nodal basin.

- Leong's pearl: The SLN is usually found beneath the clavipectoral fascia. Use tunneling dissection technique without raising flaps to the fascia and incise it. Harvest the SLN guided by a hand-held gamma probe and/or blue lymphatics.

- Digital exploration should always be done prior to the completion of selective sentinel lymphadenectomy to make sure that no suspicious or enlarged lymph nodes are retained in the surgical bed as blue dye or radiocolloid may not enter a grossly metastatic lymph node.

* Most of the pearls are extracted from Dr. Cox's chapter in Surgical Clinics of North America [Cox 2000].

REFERENCES

Albo D, Wayne JD, Hunt KK, et. al. Anaphylactic reactions to isosulfan blue dye during sentinel lymph node biopsy for breast cancer. American Journal of Surgery 2001;182(4):393-8

American Society of Breast Surgeons. Revised Consensus Statement on Guidelines for Performance of Sentinel Lymhpadenectomy for Breast Cancer [bulletin]. August 25, 2000

Barnwell JM, Arrendonodo, MA, Kollmorgen D, et al. Sentinel lymph node biopsy in breast cancer. Annals of Surgical Oncology 1998;5(2):126-130

Beahrs O, et al. Manual for Staging of Cancer. 4th ed. Philadelphia: Lippincott; 1992.

Bland KI. Enhancing the accuracy for predictors of axillary nodal metastasis in T1 carcinoma of the breast: Role of selective biopsy with lymphatic mapping. Journal of the American College of Surgeons 1996;183(3):262-4

Borgstein PJ, Pijpers R, Comans EF, et al. Sentinel lymph node biopsy in breast cancer: guidlines and pitfalls of lymphoscintigraphy and gamma probe detection. Journal of the American College of Surgeons 1998;186(3):275-283

Borgstein PJ, Meijer S, Pijpers R. Intradermal blue dye to identify sentinel lymph-node in breast cancer. Lancet 1997;349(9066):1668-9

Cabanes P, Salmon RJ, Vilcoq JR, et al. Value of axillary dissection in addition to lumpectomy and radiotherapy in early brest cancer. Lancet 1992;329(8804):1245-1248

Cady B. Lymph node metastases. Indicators, but not governors of survival. Archives of Surgery 1984;119(9):1067-72

Carter C, Alan C, Henson DE. Relation of tumor size, lymph node status and survival in 24,740 breast cancer cases. Cancer 1989;63(1):181-7

Cox CE, Salud CJ, Harrinton MA. The Role of Selective Sentinel Node Dissection in Breast Cancer. In: Leong SPL, Wong JH, editors. The Surgical Clinics of North America: Sentinel Lymph Nodes in Human Solid Cancer. Philadelphia: WB Saunders, 2000; 80(6):1759-1777

Cox CE, Bass SS, Boulware D, et al. Implementation of New Surgical Technology: Outcome Measures for Lymphatic Mapping of Breast Carcinoma. Annals of Surgical Oncology 1999;6(6):553-561

Cox CE, Pendas S, Cox JM, et al. Guidelines for sentinel node biopsy and lymphatic mapping of patients with breast cancer. Annals of Surgery 1998;227(5):645-51; discussion 651-3

Cancer Research Campaign Working Party. Cancer research campaign trial for early breast cancer. Lancet 1980;11:55-60

Fisher B, Redmond C, Poisson R, et al. Eight year results of a randomized clinical trial comparing total mastectomy and lumpectomy with and without irradiation in the treatment of breast cancer. New England Journal of Medicine 1989;320(13):822-828

Fisher B, Redmond C, Fisher ER, et al. Ten year results of randomized clinical trial comparing radical mastectomy and total mastectomy with or without radiation. New England Journal of Medicine 1985;312(11):674-682

Fisher B, Wolmark N, Bauer M, et al. The accuracy of clinical nodal staging and of limited axillary dissection as a determinant of histological nodal status in carcinoma of the breast. Surgery, Gynecology and Obstetrics 1981;152(6):765-72

Giuliano AE. See One, Do Twenty-Five, Teach One: the implementation of Sentinel Node Dissection in Breast Cancer. Annals of Surgical Oncology 1999a;6:520-521

Giuliano AE. Mapping a pathway for axillary staging: a personal perspective on the current status of sentinel lymph node dissection for breast cancer. Archives of Surgery 1999b;134(2):195-9

Giuliano AE. Intradermal Blue Dye to Identify Sentinel Lymph Node in Breast Cancer. Lancet 1997a;350(9082):958

Giuliano AE, Jones RC, Brennan M, et al. Sentinel lymphadenectomy in breast cancer. Journal of Clinical Oncology 1997b;15(6):2345-50

Giuliano AE, Kirgan DM, Guenther JM, et al. Lymphatic mapping and sentinel lymphadenectomy for breast cancer. Annals of Surgery 1994;220(3):391-8; discussion 398-401

Grant RN, Tabah EJ, Adair FE. The surgical significance of the subareolar plexus in cancer of the breast. Surgery 1959;33:71-78

Guenther JM, Krishnamoorthy M, Tan LR. Sentinel lymphadenectomy for breast cancer in a community managed care setting. Cancer Journal 1997;3(6):336-40

Haagensen CD, Feind CR, Herter FP, et al. The Lymphatics in Cancer. Philadelphia: WB Saunders; 1972.

Harlow SP, Krag DN, Weaver DL, et al. Extra-Axillary Sentinel Lymph Nodes in Breast Cancer. Breast Cancer 1999;6:159-165

Hayward J. The surgeon's role in primary breast cancer. Breast Cancer Research and Treatment 1981;1:27-32

Ivens D, Hoe AL, Podd TJ, et al. Assessment of morbidity from complete axillary dissection. British Journal of Cancer 1992;66(1):136-138

Kern KA, Rosenberg RJ. Preoperative Lymphoscintigraphy During Lymphatic Mapping for Breast Cancer: Improved Sentinel Node Imaging Using Subareolar Injection of Technetium 99m Sulfur Colloid. Journal of the American College of Surgeons 2000;191:479-489

Klimberg VS, Rubio IT, Henry R, et al. Subareolar versus peritumoral injection for location of the sentinel lymph node. Annals of Surgery 1999;229(6):860-4; discussion 864-5

Kowalsky RJ, Perry JR. Radiopharmaceuticals in Nuclear Medicine Practice. Los Altos: Appleton and Lange, 1987. p.271-314.

Krag D. The Sentinel Node for Staging Breast Cancer: Current Review. Breast Cancer 1999;6:233-236

Krag D, Weaver D, Ashikaga T, et al. The sentinel node in breast cancer--a multicenter validation study. New England Journal of Medicine 1998;339(14):941-6

Krag DN, Weaver DL, Alex JC, et al. Surgical resection and radiolocalization of the sentinel lymph node in breast cancer using a gamma probe. Surgical Oncology 1993;2(6):335-9; discussion 340

Langlands AO, Prescott RJ, Hamilton T. A clinical trial in the management of operable breast cancer. British Journal of Surgery 1980;67(3):170-174

Leong SPL, Morita ET, Treseler PA, et al. Multidisciplinary Approach to Selective Sentinel Lymph Node Mapping in Breast Cancer. Breast Cancer 2000a;7(2):105-113

Leong SPL, Donegan E, Heffernon W, et al. Adverse reactions to isosulfan blue during selective sentinel lymph node dissection in melanoma. Annals of Surgical Oncology 2000b;7:361-6

Leong SPL, Steinmetz I, Habib FA, et al. Optimal selective sentinel lymph node dissection in primary malignant melanoma. Archives of Surgery 1997;132(6):666-73; discussion 673

Linehan DC, Hill AD, Tran KN, et al. Sentinel lymph node biopsy in breast cancer: unfiltered radioisotope is superior to filtered. Journal of the American College of Surgeons 1999;188(4):377-81

McArdle CS, Crawford D, Dykes EH, et al. Adjuvant radiotherapy and chemotherapy in breast cancer. British Journal of Surgery 1986;73(4):264-6

McMasters KM, Wong SL, Martin RC 2d, et al. Dermal injection of radioactive colloid is superior to peritumoral injection for breast cancer sentinel lymph node biopsy: results of a multiinstitutional study. Annals of Surgery 2001;233:676-687

Morton DL, Wen DR, Wong JH. Technical details of intraoperative lymphatic mapping for early stage melanoma. Archives of Surgery 1992;127(4):392-9

Neiweg OEK, Peterse JL, et al. Identification of sentinel node in patients with breast carcinoma. Ned Tijdschr Geneeskd 1996;140:2235-39

Nemoto T, Vana J, Bedwani RN, et al. Management and survival of female breast cancer: Results of a national survery by the American College of Surgeons. Cancer 1980;45(12):2917-24

NIHCC. NIoHCc: Treatment of early breast cancer. JAMA 1991;265:391-5

O'Hea BHA, Hill AD, El-Shirbiny AM, et al. Sentinel lymph node biopsy in breast cancer: initial experience at Memorial Sloan-Kettering Cancer [see comments]. Journal of the American College of Surgeons 1998;186(4):423-427

Orr RK. The impact of prophylactic axillary node dissection on breast cancer survival – a Bayesian meta-analysis. Annals of Surgical Oncology 1999;6(1):109-116

Overgaard M, Hansen PS, Overgaard J, et al. Postoperative radiotherapy in high-risk premenopausal women with breast cancer who receive adjuvant chemotherapy. New England Journal of Medicine 1997;337(14):949-955

Pijpers R, Meijer S, Hoekstra OS, et al. Impact of lymphoscintigraphy on sentinel node identification with technetium-99m-colloidal albumin in breast cancer. Journal of Nuclear Medicine 1997;38(3):366-8

Ragaz J, Jackson SM, Le N, et al. Adjuvant radiotherapy and chemotherapy in node-positive premenopausal women with breast cancer. New England Journal of Medicine 1997;337(14):956-962

Roumen RM, Geuskens LM, Valkenburg JG. In search of the true sentinel node by different injection techniques in breast cancer patients. European Journal of Surgical Oncology 1999;25(4):347-51

Rouviere H. Anatomie des Lymphatiques de l'Homme. Paris: Masson, 1932.

Rutquist L, Petterson D, Johansson H. Adjuvant radiation therapy versus surgery alone in operable breast cancer; long-term follow-up in a randomized clinical trial. Radiotherapy and Oncology 1993;104:26

Sappey MPC. Anatomie, physiologie, pathologie des vaisseaux lymphatiques consideres chez l'homme et les vertebres. Paris, DeLahaye A, Lecrosnier, 1874.

Schneebaum SSY, Cohen M, et al. Sentinel lymph node localization in breast cancer- A feasibility study. Presented SSO meeting in Atlanta, GA, 1996.

Turner RR, Ollila DW, Krasne DL, et al. Histopathologic validation of the sentinel lymph node hypothesis for breast carcinoma. Annals of Surgery 1997;226(3):271-6

Turner-Warwick RT. The lymphatics of the breast. British Journal of Surgery 1953;46:574-82

Vendrell-Torne E, Setoain-Quinquer, Domenech-Torne FM. Study of Normal Mammary Lymphatic Drainage Using Radiotracer Isotopes. Journal of Nuclear Medicine 1972;13(11):801-805

Veronesi U, Paganelli G, Galimberti V, et al. Sentinel-node biopsy to avoid axillary dissection in breast cancer with clinically negative lymph nodes. Lancet 1997;349(9069):1864-7

White R, Vezeridis MP, Konstadoulakis M, et al. Therapeutic options and results for the management of minimally invasive carcinoma of the breast; influence of axillary dissection for treatment of T1a and T1b lesions. Journal of the American College of Surgeons 1996;183(6):575-522

5 PATHOLOGIC EXAMINATION OF THE SENTINEL LYMPH NODE

Patrick A. Treseler, MD, PhD

INTRODUCTION

Selective sentinel lymph node dissection is an extremely powerful technique to predict whether a malignant neoplasm has metastasized to regional lymph nodes. If the first, or sentinel, lymph node (SLN) to receive drainage from a tumor is found to be negative for metastatic tumor, numerous studies have shown the likelihood of other lymph nodes in that group containing tumor to be quite small [Albertini 1996, Bass 1999, Blaheta 1999, Borgstein 1998, Burak 1999, Crossin 1998, Cserni 1999, Czerniecki 1999, Dale 1998, Fisher 1978, Flett 1998, Giuliano 1997, Giuliano 1994, Guenther 1997, Hill 1999, Jaderborg 1999, Joseph 1999, Kelemen 1999, Kelley 1999, Koller 1998, Krag 1998, Morton 1993, Morton 1992, Offodile 1998, O'Hea 1998, Pijpers 1997, Reintgen 1994, Rubio 1998, Thompson 1995, Turner 1997, Veronesi 1997, Veronesi 1999, Wells 1997, Winchester 1999], with the false negative rate (expressed as false negatives out of all positives [McMasters 1998]) averaging about 4% in melanoma patients (Table 1), and 7% in patients with breast cancer (Table 2). Given that many patients with low stage primary tumors will have no regional nodal metastases, the number of cases in which tumor will actually be left behind in a node group from which only a negative sentinel lymph node is excised will be much lower than the theoretical false negative rates cited above

Table 1. Sentinel Lymph Node Biopsy in Melanoma Studies Comparing Full Regional Node Dissection *

Studies	Patients	Positive SLNs (%)	False-Negative Rate (%)
Morton, et al. [1992]	194	40/194 (21)	2/42 (5)
Morton, et al. [1993]	89	13/89 (15)	0/13 (0)
Reintgen, et al. [1994]	42	8/42 (19)	0/8 (0)
Thompson, et al. [1995]	105	22/105 (21)	2/24 (8)
Wells, et al. [1997]	55	6/55 (11)	0/6 (0)
Keleman, et al. [1999]	47	11/47 (23)	0/11 (0)
Joseph, et al. [1999]	127	12/127 (9)	0/12 (0)
Blaheta, et al. [1999]	73	13/73 (18)	1/14 (7)
Total	*732*	*125/732 (17)*	*5/130 (4)*

* Adapted from Treseler PA, Tauchi , PS [Treseler 2000]

Table 2. Sentinel Lymph Node Biopsy in Breast Cancer Studies Comparing Full Axillary Dissection *

Studies	Patients	Positive SLNs (%)	False-Negative Rate (%)
Giuliano, et al. [1994]	114	37/114 (32)	5/42 (12)
Albertini, et al. [1996]	57	18/57 (32)	0/18 (0)
Giuliano, et al. [1997]	100	42/100 (42)	0/42 (0)
Turner, et al. [1997]	103	43/103 (42)	1/44 (2)
Guenther, et al. [1997]	103	28/103 (27)	3/31 (10)
Pijpers, et al. [1997]	34	11/34 (32)	0/11 (0)
Veronesi, et al. [1997]	160	81/160 (51)	4/85 (5)
Dale, et al. [1998]	14	4/14 (36)	0/4 (0)
O'Hea, et al. [1998]	55	20/55 (36)	3/23 (13)
Borgestein, et al. [1998]	104	44/104 (42)	1/45 (2)
Offodile, et al. [1998]	41	18/41 (44)	0/18 (0)
Flett, et al. [1998]	56	18/56 (32)	3/21 (14)
Koller, et al. [1998]	96	35/96 (36)	3/38 (8)
Crossin, et al. [1998]	42	7/42 (17)	1/8 (12)
Krag, et al. [1998]	405	101/405 (25)	13/114 (11)
Veronesi, et al. [1999]	371	168/371 (45)	12/180 (7)
Bass, et al. [1999]	173	53/173 (31)	1/54 (2)
Rubio, et al. [1999]	53	15/53 (28)	2/17 (12)
Jaderborg, et al. [1999]	64	19/64 (30)	1/20 (5)
Cserni, et al. [1999]	58	36/58 (62)	3/39 (8)
Kelley, et al. [1999]	23	9/23 (39)	0/9 (9)
Burak, et al. [1990]	45	14/45 (31)	0/14 (0)
Winchester, et al. [1999]	162	44/162 (27)	4/48 (8)
Hill, et al. [1999]	104	47/104 (45)	5/52 (10)
Czerniecki, et al. [1999]	41	15/41 (37)	0/15 (0)
Total	*2,578*	*927/2,578 (17)*	*65/992 (7)*

* Adapted from Treseler PA, Tauchi , PS [Treseler 2000]

(which are correctly derived only from cases in which regional nodal metastases are present [McMasters 1998]. Such data have led some authorities to advocate excision of the sentinel lymph node alone as adequate assessment of the regional lymph nodes in some cancer patients [Morton 1999], sparing them the morbidity associated with a full regional node dissection [Cabanes 1992, Ivens 1992, Keramopoulos 1993, Kissin 1986, Larson 1986, Schrenk 2000].

There are two major factors involved in the high predictive value of the SLN dissection technique. The first is the specialized techniques employed by nuclear medicine physicians and surgeons to accurately identify and remove the actual first lymph node (or nodes) to receive direct lymphatic drainage from the region of a tumor. These techniques are discussed at length in other chapters in this volume. The second factor, which is likely of equal importance, is that the identification of a single sentinel lymph node (or, at most, a few sentinel nodes) permits more detailed pathologic analysis of the sentinel lymph node than would be feasible with the dozens of nodes typically identified in a full regional dissection.

These factors involved in the pathologic examination of the SLNs will be the focus of this chapter.

THE SEARCH FOR METASTATIC TUMOR IN REGIONAL LYMPH NODES

Malignant tumor cells that have gained access to the lymphatic system may drain via the normal flow of lymph to the regional lymph nodes [Foster 1996]. Tumor cells typically enter the node via the afferent lymphatic vessels, which drain into the node's subcapsular sinus [Foster 1996]. Early deposits of metastatic tumor are thus often identified in the subcapsular sinus, but tumor cells may continue to drain through the trabecular sinuses of the node cortex and medullary nodal sinuses, and may eventually leave the node via the hilar efferent lymphatic vessels to give rise to distant metastases. Tumor cells in any of these sites may lodge there and give rise to large metastatic deposits [Foster 1996].

Traditionally, pathologic examination of potentially diseased tissue has consisted of microscopic examination of a single hemtoxylin-and-eosin (H&E)-stained 5 micron (μ) tissue section cut from the formalin-fixed, paraffin-embedded tissue block. If a lymph node from a regional node dissection measured greater than 5 mm in thickness, the node would traditionally be sectioned at intervals of 5 mm of less (to permit adequate penetration of the formalin fixative), with typically only a single 5 μ histologic section submitted for microscopic analysis. The number of 5 μ histologic sections that can be cut from even a single 5 mm tissue section is quite large (approximately 1000, by simple arithmetic), with up to several thousand sections possible from a large lymph node. A regional lymph node dissection (which may contain dozens of large nodes) could in theory yield tens of thousands of histologic sections, making microscopic examination of all tissue from regional node dissections highly impractical. A single representative H&E-stained 5μ section has thus served for generations as the pathologic standard-of-care for the histologic examination of most excised tissues.

THE ADDED VALUE OF EXAMINATION OF MULTIPLE DEEPER LEVEL SECTIONS

This system of representative histologic examination of a single H&E-stained section has obvious limitations, however, if one is seeking to identify small deposits of metastatic tumor in a lymph node. It was known even in the pre-SLN era, that axillary lymph nodes from breast cancer patients may harbor metastases not evident in initial H&E-stained sections (Figure 1, Figure 2), and that examination of additional sections cut from multiple deeper levels of the axillary node paraffin blocks will identify so-called "occult" metastases in 9% to 33% of cases [Dowlatshahi 1997]. For example, data from the International (Ludwig) Breast Cancer Study Group, reported by Goldhirsch [1990], demonstated that 9% of breast

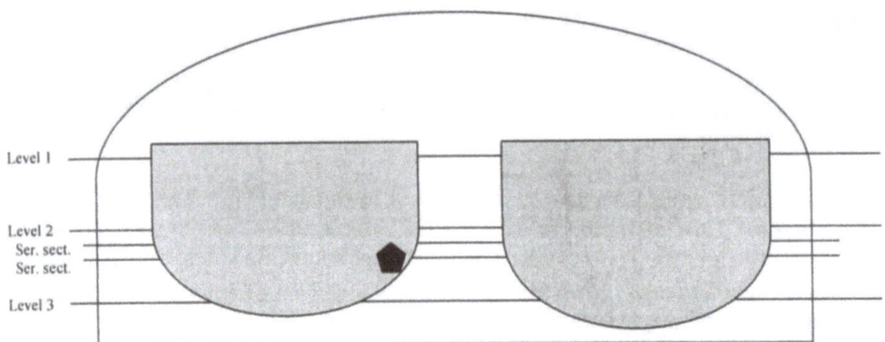

Figure 1. Deeper level sections and serial sections used to analyze a paraffin-embedded tissue block. A small metastatic deposit represented by the dark pentagon would not be identified in sections taken from just the first level.

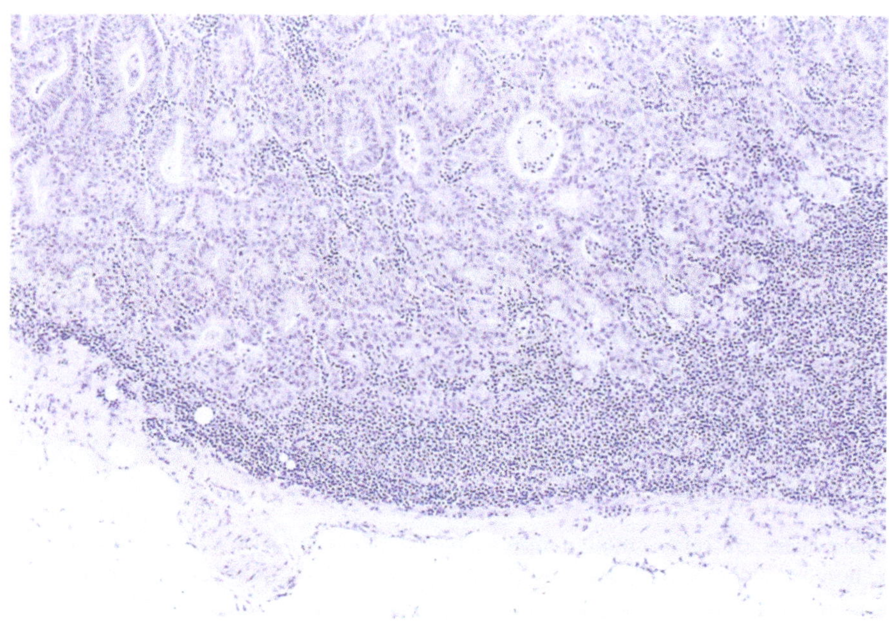

Figure 2. This small deposit of metastatic carcinoma in a sentinel lymph node from a breast cancer patient was found only in sections taken from the third level of the paraffin-embedded tissue block. No tumor was evident in the sections taken from the first or section levels. (H&E stain, original magnification 400X)

cancer patients whose axillary lymph nodes were thought to be tumor-negative by routine histologic examination were found to harbor occult tumor in those nodes when multiple deeper level H&E-stained sections of the lymph node blocks were examined. Moreover, these patients were found in retrospect to have significantly higher rates of tumor recurrence and mortality than the other patients, testifying to the clinical significance of these occult metastatic deposits [Goldhirsch 1990] (Figure 3).

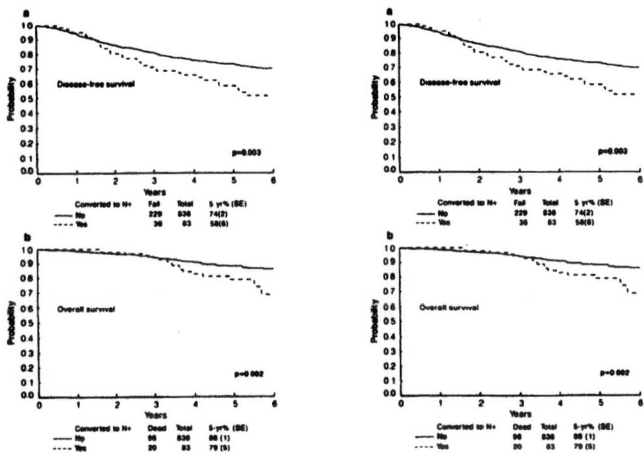

Figure 3. Disease-free (a) and overall (b) survival for 921 node-negative breast cancer patients whose axillary lymph nodes were subjected to H&E staining at multiple deeper level sections. Dashed line: Converted from node-negative to node-positive. Solid line: Remained node-negative. From Goldhirsch A, Castiglione M. Prognostic importance of occult axillary lymph node micrometastases from breast cancers. International (Ludwig) Breast Cancer Study Group [see comments]. Lancet 1990;335:1565-8, with permission.

Numerous other studies have confirmed these findings [Dowlatshahi 1997]. However, the large number of sections required to perform such analyses in full regional node dissections prevented their widespread use. With the advent of the technique of selective excision of the sentinel lymph node, however, the examination of multiple deeper level sections became much more practical, since only one (or, at most, a few) nodes from any one node group required such detailed attention. Recent studies of sentinel lymph nodes in breast cancer patients have confirmed the usefulness of multiple deeper level H&E-stained sections in the detection of occult sentinel lymph node metastases [Jannink 1998, Kelley 1999].

It is important to distinguish between *occult metastases* (as defined above, which can be of any size), the clinical significance of which is well established (at least in breast cancer patients); and *micrometastases* (a term without a clear definition), the clinical significance of which remains somewhat controversial. The term micrometastasis has been used by various authors to describe small deposits of metastatic tumor in regional lymph nodes, generally in breast cancer patients) [Fleming 1997, Huvos 1971, Nasser 1993, Sobin 1997]. The most commonly used definition of a micrometastasis is a metastatic deposit 2 mm in greatest dimension; others, however, have applied the term to various smaller deposits (down to as small as 0.2 mm in greatest dimension) [Fleming 1997, Huvos 1971, Nasser 1993, Sobin 1997]. Still others have defined the term on the basis of the percentage of the cross-sectional area of the lymph node involved by tumor [Black 1980]. Not surprisingly, these studies have varied in their conclusions concerning the significance of such microscopic tumor deposits. Nonetheless at least some studies have shown a significantly worse prognosis in patients with lymph node micrometastases, even as small as 0.5 mm [Clayton 1993, de Mascarel 1992, Nasser 1993, Rosen 1981]. Unlike micrometastases, occult metastases may be quite large [Goldhirsch 1990] (Figure 4).

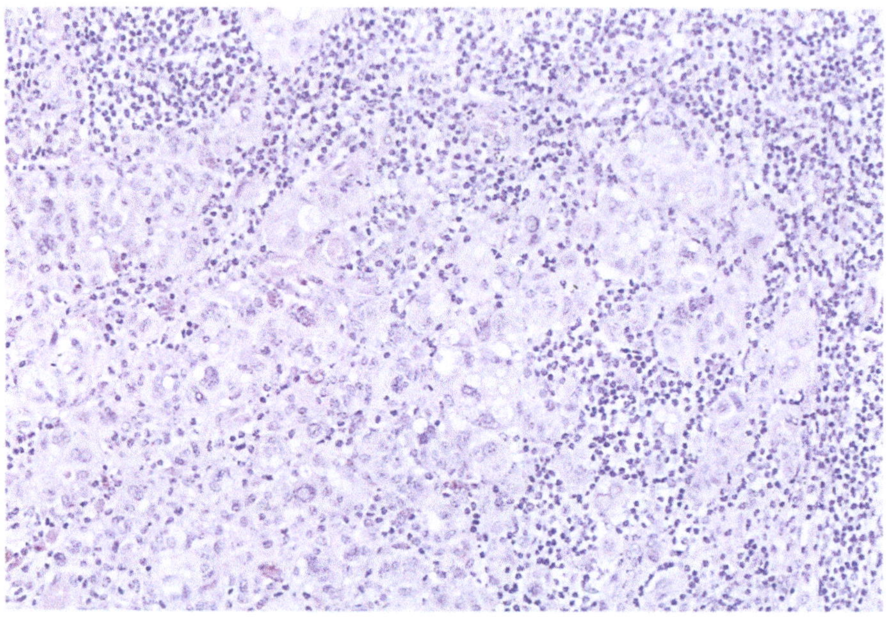

Figure 4. This large deposit of metastatic melanoma in a sentinel lymph node was found only in sections taken from the third level of the paraffin-embedded tissue block. No tumor was evident in the sections taken from the first or section levels. (H&E stain, original magnification 200X)

THE ADDED VALUE OF IMMUNOHISTOCHEMICAL STAINS

Immunoperoxidase stains for antigens relatively specific for tumor cells (such as keratin proteins or epithelial membrane antigen (EMA) for carcinoma, and S-100 or HMB-45 for melanoma) also appear to increase the yield of metastasis detection in sentinel lymph nodes. As with the use of multiple deeper level stained sections, the value of immunohistochemical stains in the detection of occult nodal metastases had been recognized even before the era of sentinel lymph node dissection. In 1993, Hainsworth and colleagues studied 343 apparently node-negative breast cancer patients [Hainsworth 1993]. With deeper level H&E-stained sections occult metastases were found in 10 patients, but 31 more occult metastases were identified by immunohistochemistry. Patients with occult metastases detected by either method had a worse prognosis. In a follow-up study of the International (Ludwig) Breast Cancer Study Group patients, reported by Cote et al. in 1999 [Cote 1999], a single unstained slide taken from the first deeper level of the lymph node block (which had been held in storage for nearly 10 years) was stained for keratin proteins. A full 20% of the patients thought to be node-negative (after H&E

examination of deeper level sections) were found, in truth, to contain metastatic carcinoma in their axillary lymph nodes after the keratin stains were examined. This group was found to have a significantly worse prognosis than those patients who remained node-negative [Cote 1999].

Several studies have now been conducted in sentinel lymph node patients to validate the usefulness of immunohistochemical stains in detecting occult metastases (Table 3). In studies of melanoma patients, the addition of immunohistochemical stains for various melanoma-associated antigens converted an average of 7% of apparently node-negative patients to node-positive [Goscin 1999, Messina 1999, Morton 1992, Morton 1993] (Table 3). In breast cancer patients, this conversion rate was even higher, with an average of 11% of patients whose nodes appeared negative for tumor by routine H&E stains being found to have nodal metastases when stains for epithelial markers were employed [Czerniecki 1999, Giuliano 1997, Kelley 1999, McIntosh 1999, Pendas 1999, Schreiber 1999, Turner 1997] (Table 3).

Table 3. Sentinel Lymph Node Metastases Detected by Hematoxylin-Eosin vs. Immunohistochemistry Staining *

	Sentinel Lymph Node Metastases Identified			
Patients	Total (%)	H&E (%)	IHC (%)	IHC Conversion Rate ** %
Melanoma Studies				
Morton, et al. [1992] 194	40 (21)	23 (12)	17 (9)	10
Morton, et al. [1993] 89	13 (15)	8 (9)	5 (6)	6
Goscin, et al. [1999] 405	72 (18)	50 (12)	22 (5)	6
Messina, et al. [1999] 357	56 (16)	31 (9)	25 (7)	8
Total 1045	*181 (17)*	*112 (11)*	*69 (7)*	*7*
Breast Cancer Studies				
Giuliano, et al. [1997] 100	42 (42)	33 (33)	9 (9)	13
Turner, et al. [1997] 103	43 (42)	33 (32)	10 (10)	14
Schreiber, et al. [1999] 210	47 (22)	30 (14)	17 (8)	9
Pendas, et al. [1999] 478	134 (28)	93 (19)	41 (9)	11
Czerniecki, et al. [1999] 41	15 (37)	12 (29)	3 (7)	10
Kelley, et al. [1999] 28	9 (32)	8 (29)	1 (4)	5
McIntosh, et al. [1999] 116	72 (62)	64 (55)	8 (7)	15
Total 1076	*362 (34)*	*273 (25)*	*89 (8)*	*11*

* Adapted from Treseler PA, Tauchi , PS [Treseler 2000]
** Percentage of cases negative by H&E stain that converted to positive with IHC staining.

The benefit of immunohistochemical stains appears to derive mainly from their ability to detect tumor deposits that are either too small or too cytologically bland to be readily detected in routine H&E-stained sections [Cote 1999]. The majority of nodal metastases of breast cancer or melanoma produce deposits of metastatic tumor that are easily identified in H&E-stain sections (Figure 5).

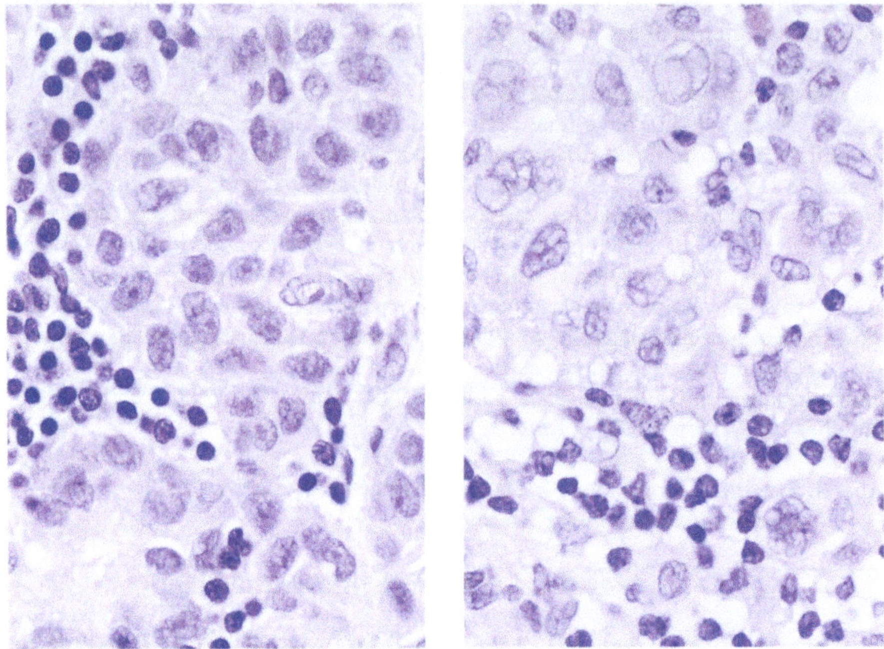

Figure 5. Metastatic ductal breast cancer (A) and melanoma (B) in sentinel lymph nodes from separate patients. These tumors are typical nodal metastases in that they display prominent cytologic atypia, and can be detected in routine H&E-stained tumor sections. (H&E stain, original magnification 200X)

However, a significant minority may be quite cytologically bland. Invasive lobular breast cancer, for example, is composed of relatively bland small round cells. Detection of such cells is difficult even in primary breast biopsies, where the small blue tumor cells contrast against the pink fibrous breast stroma in routine H&E-stained sections (Figure 6a). Even better camouflage is provided these tumor cells by the small round blue lymphocytes that predominate in an H&E-stained lymph node (Figure 6b). Keratin stains performed on such lymph nodes may reveal extensive infiltration by lobular carcinoma cells, despite a virtually normal appearance in the H&E-stained sections (Figure 6c). For example, in the report of Ludwig Study breast cancer patients by Cote et al. described above, the majority of the many patients found to have occult sentinel lymph node metastases by keratin staining had invasive lobular breast cancer [Cote 1999]. Similarly, melanoma cells (which are renowned for their ability to mimic a wide variety of benign and malignant cells, including sinus histiocytes of lymph nodes (Figure 7) may be virtually impossible to detect in some sentinel lymph nodes without special stains [Charny 1995, Cochran 2000] (Figure 8).

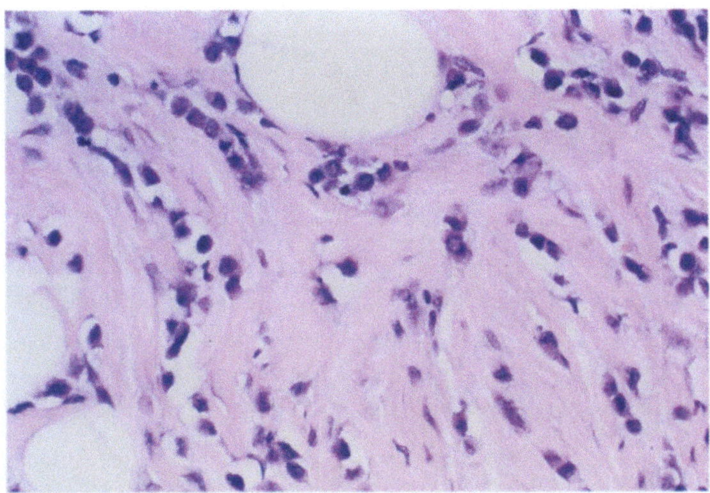

Figure 6a. Invasive lobular breast cancer. Primary lobular in the breast. Tumor cells are small and relatively monomorphic, but can be recognized as invasive carcinoma due to characteristic single file infiltration of tumor cells through lighter staining fibrous stroma (H&E stain, original magnification 1000X).

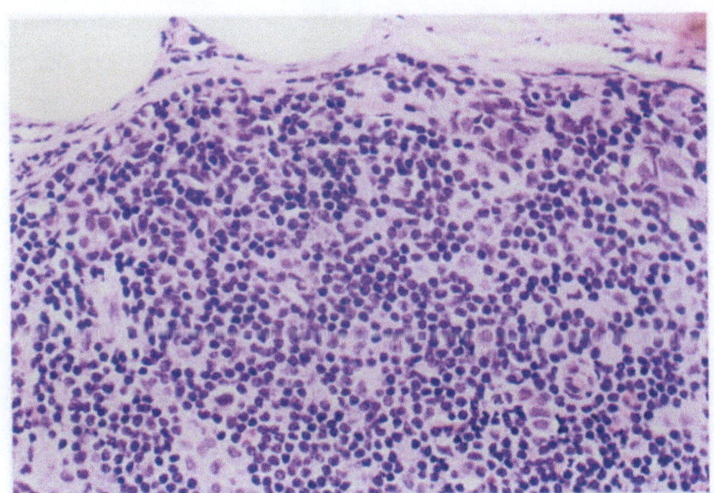

Figure 6b. Invasive lobular breast cancer. Metastatic lobular carcinoma in sentinel lymph node. Tumor cells are numerous in the field (e.g., cluster in upper right), but are nearly perfectly camouflaged by the numerous surrounding small lymphocytes. (H&E stain, original magnification 1000X).

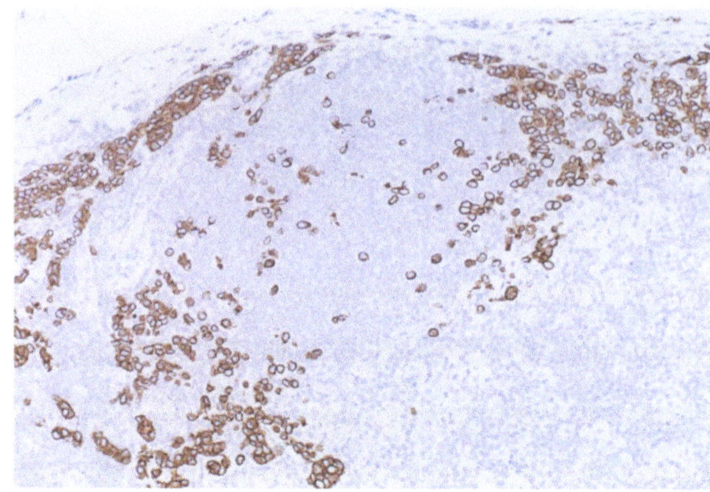

Figure 6c. Invasive lobular breast cancer. Metastatic lobular carcinoma in sentinel lymph node. A keratin immunoperoxidase stain highlights the numerous tumor cells. (AE1/3 and CAM5.2 Keratin immunoperoxidase stain, original magnification 400X)

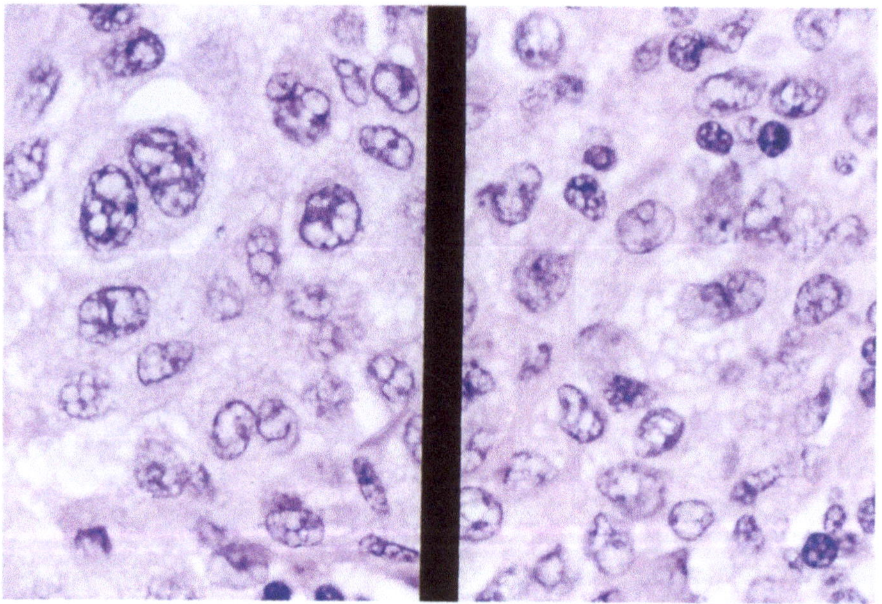

Figure 7. The mimicry of benign sinus histiocytes by melanoma cells. Left panel: Metastatic melanoma cells. Right panel: True sinus histiocytes. (H&E stain, original magnification 1000X)

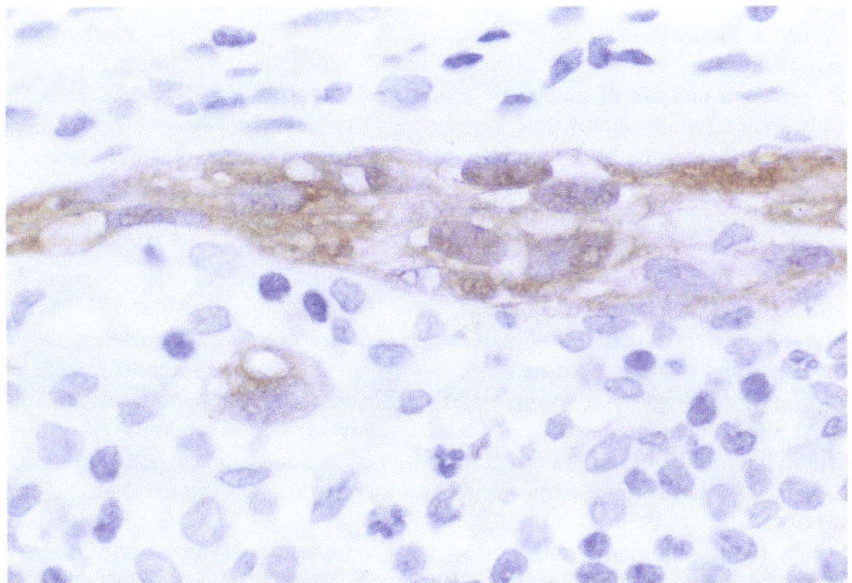

Figure 8. Metastatic melanoma in lymph node subcapsular sinus. An S-100 immunoperoxidase stain highlights the cells, which otherwise are quite bland and difficult to distinguish from sinus histiocytes. (H&E stain, original magnification 400X)

THE RISKS OF IMMUNOHISTOCHEMICAL STAINS: FALSE POSITIVES AND FALSE NEGATIVES

Immunohistochemical stains used to detect occult metastases in sentinel lymph nodes can thus be thought of as a clinical test used to screen an at-risk population for a particular disease. As with any other clinical lab test, there is the potential for false positive and false negative results, which could lead to erroneous interpretation of the stains. Luckily, the majority of these potential errors can be avoided if one understands the limitations of the various immunohistochemical stains typically employed in the evaluation of sentinel lymph nodes.

The problem of false positives and false negatives in sentinel lymph node immunohistochemistry is much more of an issue in melanoma sentinel lymph nodes than in axillary nodes from breast cancer patients. This stems from the lack of a single highly specific and highly sensitive antigen that can be used to identify melanoma cells.

Antibodies to four antigens are typically used to identify melanoma cells: S-100 protein, NK1/C3, Melan-A (also known as MART-1 (Melanoma Antigen Recognized by T-cells)), and HMB-45. But these vary widely in their sensitivity and specificity for melanoma. S-100 protein is the most sensitive marker for melanoma, expressed in close to 100% of cases [Blessing 1998, Busam 1998, Kaufmann 1998] (but it still may be entirely absent in rare melanoma cases [Kaufmann 1998]). It is quite non-specific, however, being commonly expressed by a significant proportion of carcinomas, lymphomas, sarcomas, and other neoplasms [Cochran 1993]. In normal lymph nodes, S-100 protein is strongly expressed by both follicular dendritic cells within lymphoid follicles and interfollicular interdigitating reticulum cells [Gloghini 1990, Shamoto 1993, Sudilovsky 1998]. These normal cells, which occur as individual or loosely aggregated cells with a dendritic morphology, can usually be readily distinguished from the tightly aggregated cell clusters of metastatic melanoma (Figure 9). S-100 protein is also strongly expressed by nevus cell aggregates (also called nodal nevi), which are aggregates of benign nevomelanocytic cells found in up to 9% of lymph nodes [yu 1999]. These can generally be distinguished from metastatic melanoma by the absence of cytologic atypia and mitotic activity, and by their characteristic location within the fibrous tissue of the lymph node capsule (Figure 10)[Warnke 1995]. Because nodal nevi may occasionally extend into the nodal parenchyma, and because some metastatic melanomas may be cytologically bland with low proliferative rates, the distinction may be difficult in some cases [Van Diest 1999a]. At the other end of the spectrum, HMB-45 is a marker highly specific for cells of nevomelanocytic origin (and thus may be weakly positive even in nodal nevi), but is the least sensitive, being negative in approximately 15% of melanomas [Kaufmann 1998]. In the middle of this spectrum lie the other two common melanoma markers, NK1/C3 and Melan-A, both with sensitivities and specificities intermediate between those of S-100 and HMB-45 [Bishop 1993, Blessing 1998, Fernando 1994, Jungbluth 1998, Kaufmann 1998]. Most melanoma sentinel lymph node studies to date have utilized antibodies against S-100 protein, with many utilizing anti-HMB-45 antibodies as well. A summary of the causes of false positive and false negative immunohistochemical staining results in melanoma is shown in Table 4.

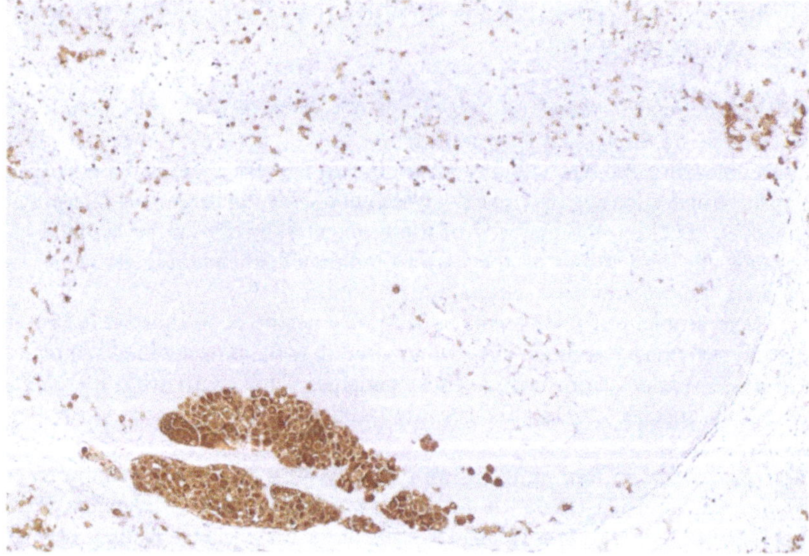

Figure 9. Melanoma sentinel lymph node with S-100 immunoperoxidase stain. The stain highlights scattered follicular dendritic cells (upper left) and interdigitating reticulum cells (lower left), but metastatic melanoma cells show characteristic darkly stained, tightly clustered cell aggregates not typical of the S-100-positive dendritic cell populations. (S-100 immunoperoxidase stain, original magnification 200X)

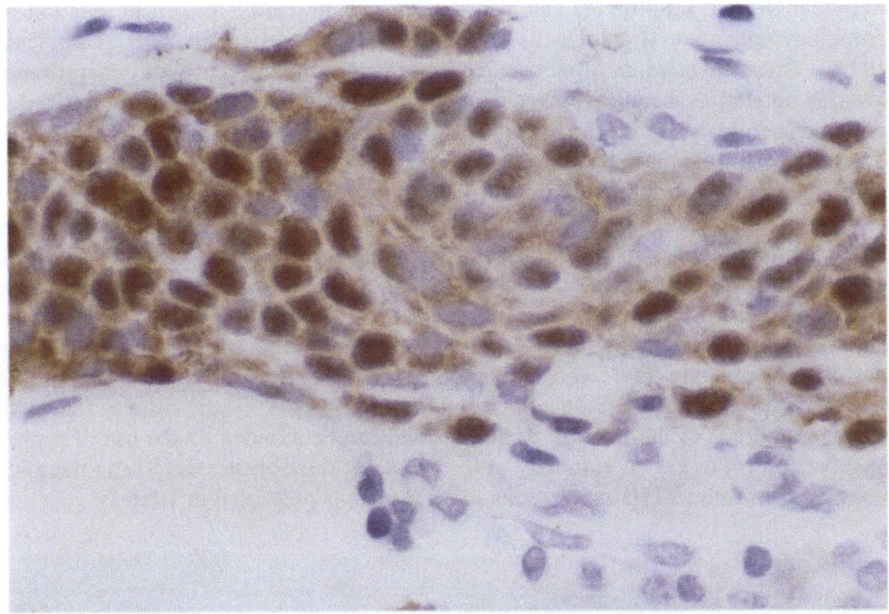

Figure 10. Nodal nevus cell aggregate. Lack of significant cytologic atypia, lack of mitotic figures, and characteristic location within the lymph node capsule distinguish this entity (which stains positively for S-100 and occasionally for HMB-45) from metastatic melanoma in most cases.   (S-100 immunoperoxidase stain, original magnification 200X)

Table 4
<u>Melanoma Immunohistochemistry: False Positives and False Negatives</u>
False Positives:
- S-100-positive metastases other than melanoma (carcinoma, sarcoma, lymphoma)
- S-100-positive normal lymph node cells (follicular dendritic cells, interdigitating reticulum cells)
- Benign nevus cell aggregates (nodal nevi, capsular nevi)

False Negatives:
- Loss of expression of S-100, Melan-A, NK1/C3, HMB-45, or other melanoma-associated antigens by metastatic melanoma
- Technical failure of stain (can be avoided by proper controls)

Most studies to date reporting use of immunoperoxidase staining in the analysis of breast sentinel lymph nodes have utilized antibodies to keratin proteins. Keratin proteins are cytoplasmic intermediate filaments quite sensitive and specific for epithelial-derived cells, particularly when so-called "pan-keratin" antibodies or antibody cocktails are used (which will, at least in theory, react with all keratin types [Frisman 1994]). The typical uniform, dark staining of metastatic carcinoma for keratin proteins is shown in Figure 11. Keratin proteins may on occasion be expressed by neoplasms other than carcinomas (e.g., 7% of melanomas may be keratin-positive), but the staining detected in such non-epithelial tumors is generally weaker and more focal [Bishop 1993].   On very high-power microscopic examination, keratin proteins can also be detected in a little-known population of normal lymph node stromal cells termed fibroblastic reticulum cells [Domagala 1992]. These cells, while often present in reactive lymph nodes, will generally not even be noticed at scanning power in a keratin-stained node, but may be noticed if one is carefully screening for metastatic lobular carcinoma at high power. Their dendritic morphology, their presence as scattered single cells throughout the entire node, and their very faint staining for keratin proteins are all clues to their proper identity [Domagala 1992]. Some studies have employed antibodies to EMA or mucin proteins, either in addition to, or instead of, anti-keratin antibodies [Cserni 1999, Kelley 1999]. However, these studies offer no evidence to indicate that these antibodies are any more sensitive or specific for epithelial cells than anti-keratin antibodies, nor that they increase the yield of sentinel lymph node metastases. False negative results are rare when cocktails of anti-keratin antibodies, capable of reacting with all keratin proteins, are used [Frisman 1994]. These usually represent technical failures of the staining technique, and can be avoided by the use of proper positive control tissue. A summary of the causes of false positive and false negative immunohistochemical staining results in carcinoma is presented in Table 5.

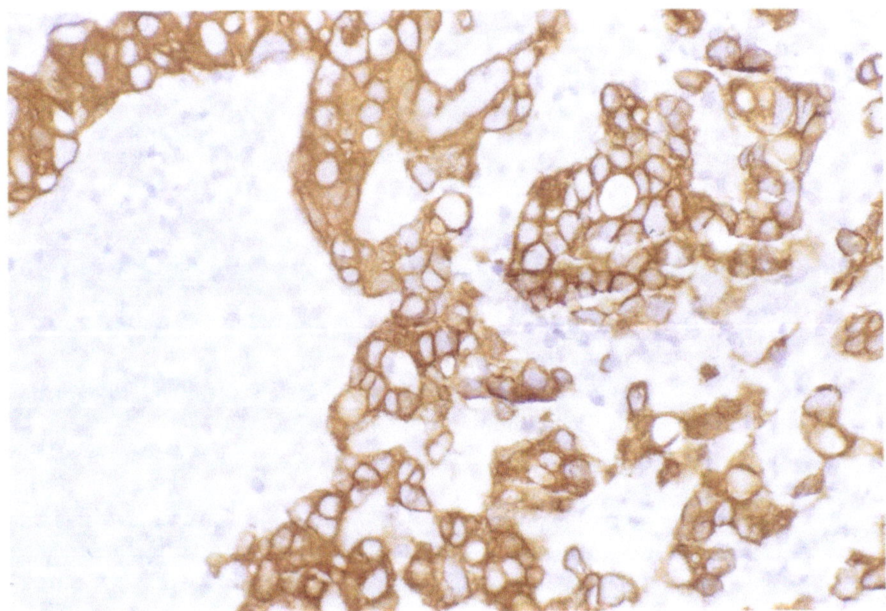

Figure 11. Metastatic ductal carcinoma in a sentinel lymph node. The uniform dark staining of the tumor cells for keratin proteins is typical of metastatic carcinoma, and would be uncommon in other keratin-positive malignancies. (AE1/3 and CAM5.2 Keratin immunoperoxidase stain, original magnification 400X)

Table 5.
Carcinoma Immunohistochemistry: False Positives and False Negatives
False Positives:
- Keratin-positive metastases other than carcinoma

- Keratin-positive normal lymph node cells (fibroblastic reticulum cells)

False Negatives:

- Insensitive anti-keratin antibodies which fail to detect some keratin proteins (can be avoided by use of antibody cocktails)
- Technical failure of stain (can be avoided by proper controls)

INTRAOPERATIVE ASSESSMENT OF THE SENTINEL LYMPH NODE: TO FREEZE OR NOT TO FREEZE?

While some surgeons continue to perform full regional node dissections after all cases of sentinel lymph node excision, others have begun to advocate sentinel lymph node biopsy as a stand-alone procedure, with completion lymphadenectomy being performed only if the sentinel lymph node is negative for tumor. Ideally, surgeons who do not perform completion lymphadenectomy routinely after sentinel lymph node excision would like to know during the procedure whether the excised node contains metastatic tumor. This would permit the surgeon to complete dissection of the entire regional node group during the same operation, eliminating the need for a second surgery. Some authorities thus advocate routine intraoperative pathologic analysis of the sentinel lymph node, particularly in cases where the patient has a primary tumor felt to be at high risk for regional nodal metastases [Van Diest 1999b, Viale 1999]. Others point out the large amount of lymph node tissue which is generally lost in "facing up" a frozen tissue block for frozen section (estimated as high as 50% of total nodal tissue [Van Diest 1999c]), the risk of false positives due to suboptimal frozen section histology, and the introduction of freeze-thaw artifact into the permanent section tissue; these authors argue against performing frozen section in most cases [Anderson 1999, Pfeifer 1999]. Intra-operative cytologic touch imprints (also referred to as touch preparations or imprint cytology) can be made without significant loss of or damage to lymph node tissue, but considerable expertise is required for proper interpretation of such cytologic preparations, which can affect diagnostic accuracy [Turner 1999a].

In addition, intra-operative assessment of sentinel lymph nodes is plagued by high false negative rates. Routine frozen section analysis of sentinel lymph node biopsies (in which one to three H&E stained sections are prepared from a bisected node) has been found in two separate studies to be falsely negative in 36% of breast cancer patients, when compared with the final pathologic interpretation of the node [Van Diest 1999c, Veronesi 1997]. Frustrated by such high false negative rates, one of these groups subsequently performed exhaustive intra-operative assessment of all breast sentinel lymph node tissue using both H&E stains and keratin immunoperoxidase stains at 30 or more levels through the entire tissue block [Veronesi 1999, Viale 1999]. While this approach does have the advantage of essentially forbidding false negatives by examining all lymph node tissue intra-operatively, it is generally regarded as too labor-intensive to be practical in most laboratories [Anderson 1999, Krag 1999]. In melanoma, the false negative rates for frozen section examination of sentinel lymph nodes in the single published study appears to be even higher, with a 71% false negative rate reported by Gibbs et al. [Gibbs 1999]. Analysis of intra-operative imprint cytology in breast sentinel lymph nodes appears even less sensitive. Van Diest et al. [1999c] found intra-operative imprint cytology to have a false negative rate of 36% (vs. 9% for traditional frozen section), while Ku [1999] found a false negative rate of 70%. Even combining imprint cytology with frozen section yielded a false negative rate of 52% in a study of breast sentinel lymph nodes by Turner and colleagues [Turner 1999a]. The one reported study of intra-operative imprint cytology in melanoma sentinel lymph nodes found a false negative rate of 37.5% [Messina 1999], a result similar to that reported by Veronesi's group [Veronesi 1997] for breast sentinel lymph nodes.

Further studies will likely be required to define the optimal role of intra-operative assessment of sentinel lymph node biopsies. For the present, whether or not to perform intra-operative pathologic assessment of a sentinel lymph node biopsy should be a joint decision between the surgeon and the pathologist based on the likelihood of metastases and the relative risks and benefits to the patient in a given case.

HOW MUCH IS ENOUGH?: OPTIMAL SAMPLING OF THE SENTINEL LYMPH NODE

The precise method by which the sentinel lymph node has been examined pathologically has varied widely in published studies. In breast cancer, literally dozens of studies describing the results of sentinel lymph node biopsy have appeared in the literature in the past decade [Albertini 1996, Bass 1999, Borgstein 1998, Burak 1999, Crossin 1998, Cserni 1999, Czerniecki 1999, Dale 1998, Flett 1998, Giuliano 1997, Giuliano 1994, Guenther 1997, Hill 1999, Jaderborg 1999, Kelley 1999, Koller 1998, Krag 1998, McIntosh 1999, Offodile 1998, O'Hea 1998, Pendas 1999, Pijpers 1997, Rubio 1998, Schreiber 1999, Turner 1997, Veronesi 1999, Veronesi 1997, Winchester 1999]. Making comparisons between these studies is difficult, because virtually all use different methods for pathologic analysis of the sentinel lymph nodes, with the method not even detailed in a distressingly large number of studies [Bass 1999, Burak 1999, Crossin 1998, Dale 1998, Flett 1998, Giuliano 1994, Jaderborg 1999, Koller 1998, O'Hea 1998]. Where stated, the methods vary widely, with some studies using just a single H&E-stained section for nodal analysis[Krag 1998, Pijpers 1997], while others take sections at up to 10 levels through the block [Winchester 1999] and/or use multiple immunoperoxidase stains [Kelley 1999] as a routine procedure.

Overall, breast cancer studies have found metastases to the sentinel lymph node in about 36% of cases (Table 2). As a general rule, the studies utilizing only routine histology have tended to find lower rates of sentinel lymph node positivity, in the range of 17% to 32% [Albertini 1996, Crossin 1998, Flett 1998, Giuliano 1994, Jaderborg 1999, Krag 1998, Pijpers 1997, Rubio 1998]. In contrast, studies utilizing immunoperoxidase stains and sectioning of blocks at multiple levels had some of the highest rates of node positivity, ranging from 42% to 62% [Borgstein 1998, Cserni 1999, Giuliano 1997, Turner 1997]. But of course these differences could also reflect other differences in the surgical or pathological technique, or patient variables such as primary tumor size. Thus few firm guidelines concerning optimal sentinel lymph node analysis can be gleaned from comparison of these studies.

More recently, however, several studies have been published that were specifically designed to address the issue of "how much is enough" in the pathologic evaluation of the sentinel lymph node in breast cancer. Several of these studies, by Turner et al. [1999b], Viale et al. [1999], and Cserni [1999] have reached very similar conclusions. In each of these studies, examination of at least three levels, cut at roughly 40 to 100 micron intervals, of a properly sectioned (at no more than 5 mm intervals) and properly oriented (to expose the maximum nodal surface area in the initial microscopic sections) identified 70% to 95% of the sentinel lymph nodes containing metastases. However, exhaustive sectioning of the tissue blocks, at 60 or more levels, was required to ensure that all sentinel lymph nodes containing metastatic tumor were identified. In the study by Turner et al., only 4% of lymph nodes (3% of patients) appearing negative for tumor after the first two levels converted to positive upon more extensive sampling. In the report published by Viale and co-workers, 64% of the sentinel lymph nodes containing metastases were properly identified in the very first level, 70% in the first two levels, and 77% in the first three levels (Figure 12). But it was necessary to go the

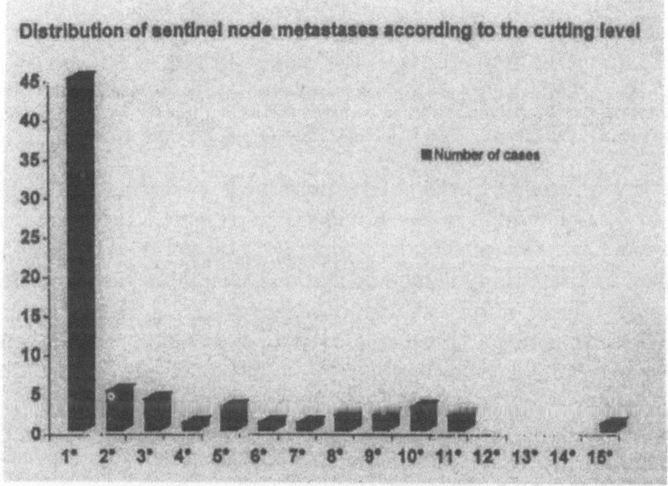

Figure 12. Levels at which metastatic carcinoma first became evident in bisected axillary sentinel lymph nodes from 70 patients with metastatic breast cancer. From: Viale G, Bosari S, Mazzarol G, et al. Intraoperative examination of axillary sentinel lymph nodes in breast carcinoma patients. Cancer 1999;85(11):2433-8, with permission.

fifteenth and final level to identify 100% of the lymph nodes with metastases. Similarly, Cserni [1999] identifed 70% of positive lymph nodes in the first microscopic level, and 75% by the fifth level. As with Viale's patients, however, the blocks had to be virtually exhausted of tissue, with sections taken at up to 45 levels through the tissue block, before 100% of the lymph nodes with metastases could be properly classified (Figure 13).

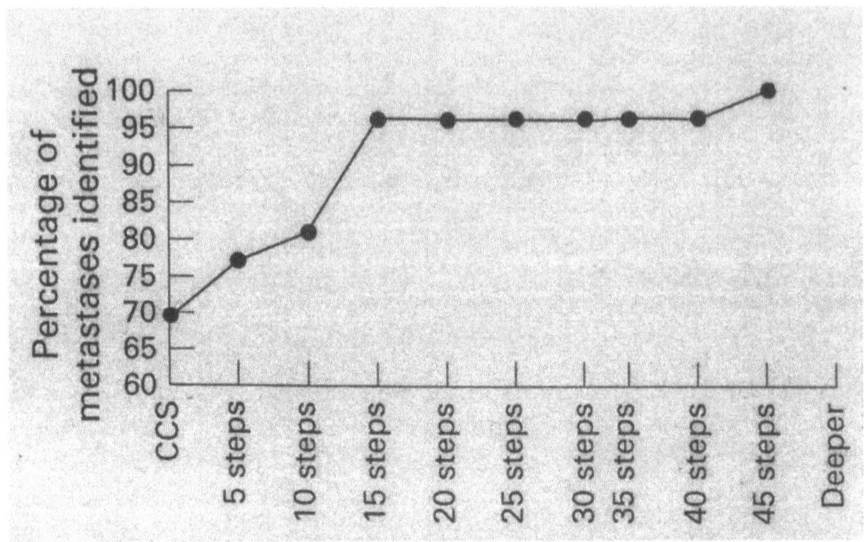

Figure 13. Number of levels (step sections) required for the identification of a given percentage of metastases in bisected sentinel lymph nodes from 58 patients with metastatic breast cancer. From: Cserni G. Metastases in axillary sentinel lymph nodes in breast cancer as detected by intensive histopathological work up [see comments]. Journal of Clinical Pathology 1999;52(12):922-924, with permission.

Far fewer studies have been published concerning the pathologic examination of sentinel lymph nodes in melanoma patients. The basic studies that proved the predictive value of sentinel lymph node biopsy in melanoma (Table 1) suffer from the same variability in method that was seen in the breast cancer studies. Some used only routine H&E staining [Thompson 1995], or did not state the method at all [Kelemen 1999]. Most employed a combination of H&E staining and immunoperoxidase staining, with the precise number of levels examined often not clearly stated [Blaheta 1999, Joseph 1999, Morton 1993, Morton 1992, Reintgen 1994, Wells 1997]. The sentinel lymph node positivity rate is lower overall in melanoma than in breast cancer, averaging about 17%, with a range of 9% to 23% in published studies (Table 1), with no clear correlation between method of pathologic analysis and sentinel lymph node positivity rate.

There are few studies in the literature concerning optimal pathologic analysis of sentinel lymph nodes in cases of malignant melanoma. Yu et al. [1999] reported that immunoperoxidase stains for S-100 protein, HMB-45, NK1/C3, and Melan-A, performed at three deeper level sections, detected metastatic melanoma in 11 of 94 cases (12%) of melanoma sentinel lymph nodes called negative on the basis of a single initial H&E-stained section. Whether routine H&E stains performed at these same levels would have detected a similar number of occult metastases cannot be determined from this study. The added value of immunohistochemistry in the detection of sentinel lymph node metastases can be inferred, however, from the four melanoma sentinel lymph node studies which have separately reported metastasis rates for H&E and immunoperoxidase stains [Goscin 1999, Messina 1999, Morton 1993, Morton 1992] (Table 3), as previously discussed.

From the above discussion, it is clear that while many gaps remain in our knowledge of optimal pathologic analysis of sentinel lymph nodes, some tentative general conclusions can be drawn. First, the traditional pathologic standard of one H&E-stained section per node appears inadequate for the analysis of sentinel lymph nodes; the examination of sections from multiple deeper levels of the node will significantly raise the number of metastases detected. Second, the addition of immunoperoxidase stains for tumor-related antigens (e.g., keratin proteins for carcinoma, S-100 and HMB-45 for melanoma) significantly increases the number of sentinel lymph node metastases detected. Third, examination of at least three levels (at approximately 40 to 100 micron intervals) of a properly bisected (or multi-sected) sentinel lymph node appears to detect somewhere between 70% and 95% of the tumor-positive sentinel lymph nodes that can be detected by deeper level sections. To detect 100% of involved nodes, however, appears to require exhaustive sectioning of the tissue blocks.

Based on such data, preliminary recommendations have been published for the pathologic handling of sentinel lymph node biopsy specimen, with the recognition that these represent "a work in progress". Cibull [1999], writing for the College of American Pathologists Surgical Pathology Committee, has recommended that the entire sentinel lymph node be submitted for pathologic evaluation, and that H&E stains be performed at three levels of the specimen block (without a particular interval depth specified), with intervening sections held on glass slides for use in immunohistochemical studies if the H&E-stained sections appear negative for tumor. Keratin stains are recommended for breast sentinel lymph nodes, and S-100 and/or HMB-45 stains for melanoma sentinel lymph nodes. This is essentially the practice followed at this author's institution, where the deeper level sections are taken at roughly 50 to 100 micron intervals (depending on the judgment of the histotechnologist regarding specimen thickness), and unstained sections are taken for possible immunohistochemistry immediately following the second H&E level. (This procedure is diagrammatically represented in Figure 14 and Figure 15). A preliminary reading of the H&E-stained sections is made immediately after staining, permitting the unstained slides to be submitted for same day immunoperoxidase staining if routine H&E-stained sections contain no evident tumor. No attempt is made to exhaust the tissue blocks, leaving tissue present for special procedures that may be developed in the future.

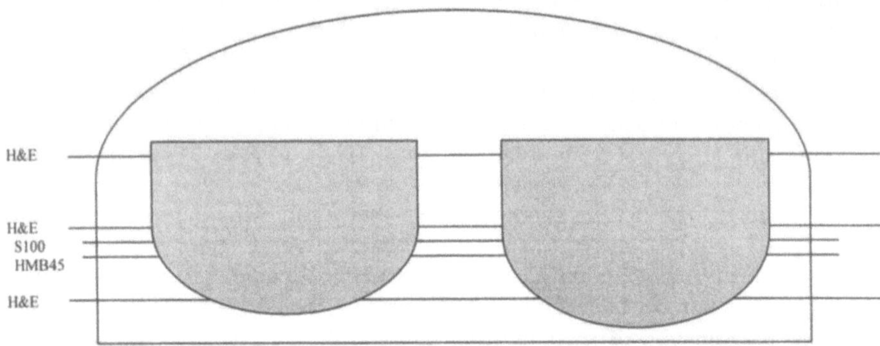

Figure 14. Proposed technique for pathologic sampling of sentinel lymph node for melanoma, which conforms to CAP recommendations. Note: For purposes of illustration, the levels are shown more widely spaced than would be typical in actual sectioning.

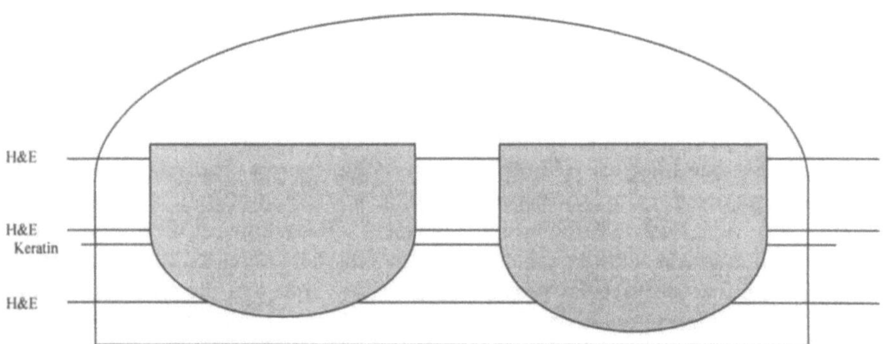

Figure 15. Proposed technique for pathologic sampling of sentinel lymph node for carcinoma, which conforms to CAP recommendations. Note: For purposes of illustration, the levels are shown more widely spaced than would be typical in actual sectioning.

A LOOK TO THE FUTURE: PCR-BASED STUDIES

The use of more sensitive methods, such as immunohistochemistry and examination of multiple deeper level sections, significantly increases the proportion of cases in which metastases to sentinel lymph nodes are found. This immediately raises the question of whether even more sensitive methods, such as those based on polymerase chain reaction (PCR), could further improve metastasis detection. Several studies have been performed to address this question.

As with any other diagnostic test, questions must be answered concerning the sensitivity and specificity of the technique (i.e., what are the risks of false positives and false negatives). Furthermore, even for true positive cases, the issue of the biological significance of the findings must be addressed before the technique can be routinely used for clinical decision-making. Just as controversy exists over the biologic significance of lymph node micrometastases, the risk imparted by a PCR-positive lymph node must be clearly understood before important clinical interventions are made.

What is clear from published studies is that PCR based assays will detect evidence of epithelial cells or nevomelanocytic cells in sentinel lymph nodes that appear negative for metastatic carcinoma or melanoma by routine H&E and immunoperoxidase stains. Schoenfeld et al. [1994] used a RT-PCR assay for keratin 19 mRNA to study sentinel lymph nodes in breast cancer patients. In their study, 15% of patients whose sentinel nodes were negative by routine H&E stains and had a positive PT-PCR reaction. Several groups have performed similar RT-PCR studies in melanoma sentinel lymph nodes, most using assays for tyrosinase mRNA [Bieligk 1999, Blaheta 1999, Hatta 1999, Joseph 1997, Lukowsky 1999, Shivers 1998, Van der Velde-Zimmermann 1996], but with one recent report looking for MART-1 and MAGE-3 mRNA as well [Bostick 1999]. These studies found positive RT-PCR reactions in 21% to 65% of patients whose sentinel lymph nodes appeared negative for tumor by routine H&E and immunohistochemical stains, with an average conversion rate of 47% based on the combined data.

What is less clear is the biological and clinical significance of sentinel lymph node whose only evidence of metastatic disease is a positive PCR reaction. To begin, it should be understood that all of the PCR studies performed in sentinel lymph nodes to date have required digestion of the assayed tissue to retrieve the mRNA for analysis. Thus, in contrast to H&E or immunohistochemical stains, there can be no morphologic assessment of the cells responsible for the positive reaction. It is therefore unclear whether the positive PCR reaction was derived from benign epithelial inclusions, benign breast epithelium passively transported into axillary lymph nodes after biopsy [Carter 2000], benign nevus cell aggregates, or even benign nerve tissue, all of which are capable of generating a positive PCR reaction [Bostick 1999]. Indeed, one PCR study of melanoma sentinel lymph nodes regarded a positive PCR signal as a false positive if there was evidence of a benign nevus cell aggregate in the tissue examined by routine stains [Blaheta 1999]. However, there was no way to determine how many of their "true positive" cases had nevus cell aggregates in the tissue digested for PCR. In addition, PCR-based assays may yield false positive results due to contamination of the samples in the laboratory. Another of the above melanoma sentinel lymph node studies found positive PCR reactions in some control lymph node tissue from patients with no history of melanoma [Bieligk 1999]. Whether such reactions were due to the presence of begin nevus cell aggregates or nerve in the control tissue, or to laboratory contamination by exogenous mRNA or DNA (another common source of false-positive reactions in PCR) is uncertain. However, it is clear that the loss in such PCR-based techniques of the ability of analyze the morphology of the cells responsible for the positive test result places some limits on the conclusions that can be drawn from such tests.

On a more mundane level, it should be noted that many studies of PCR in sentinel lymph nodes divide the sentinel node in half, with half submitted for routine H&E and immunohistochemical stains, and the other half submitted for PCR [Bieligk 1999, Blaheta 1999, Hatta 1999, Schoenfeld 1994, Shivers 1998, Van der Velde-Zimmermann 1996]. This is important because other non-PCR studies have found that the metastatic disease was present in only one half of the node in 40% of sentinel lymph node cases [Smith 1999]. Thus, it is possible that a significant proportion of "PCR-positive only" cases may simply be metastases that would have been detected by routine methods if the entire node had been submitted for routine pathologic analysis.

The best indication of clinical significance of a "PCR-positive only" sentinel lymph node would be follow-up data to suggest that this phenotype imparts a higher risk of recurrent disease. Two recent studies have produced data to indicate that such cases do have a higher risk of relapse. Shivers et al. [1998] found that melanoma relapse rates were highest (61%) in patients whose sentinel lymph node was both pathologically and PCR-positive. However, those with pathologically-negative, PCR-positive nodes had a relapse rate (13%) that, while lower than the pathologically-positive group, was significantly higher than the relapse rate seen in patients with nodes negative by both pathology and PCR (2%). Similarly, Bostick et al. [1999] found the highest recurrence rates in melanoma patients with pathologically-positive sentinel lymph nodes, but those with "PCR-positive only" nodes still had a significantly higher recurrence rate than those who were PCR-negative. In neither study did a majority of the "PCR-positive only" patients develop recurrent disease, although follow-up times were relatively short. Also, as mentioned previously, it is unknown what proportion of these cases would have revealed metastatic melanoma or benign nevus cell aggregates in the tissue used for PCR had that tissue simply been submitted for routine pathologic study.

The above data suggest that, for the present, caution should be exercised in the interpretation of positive PCR reactions where there is no morphologic evidence of metastatic disease. As a group, such patients may be at increased risk of recurrent disease, but for the individual patient it cannot even be said with certainty that the positive reaction indicates malignancy in the node. Such PCR-based assays could certainly be reasonably used to select patients who might benefit from closer clinical follow-up, but it remains unclear at present whether further therapy is warranted in such patients. This, as well as other mysteries of the sentinel lymph node, awaits further study for clarification.

CONCLUSION

The technique of sentinel lymph node biopsy has permitted accurate identification by surgeons and nuclear medicine physicians of the first node to receive direct drainage from an area of tumor. This selective dissection of the first draining node has had the added benefit of dramatically reducing the number of nodes the pathologist must examine in the search for metastatic tumor. This in turn has made feasible the routine examination of multiple levels of the submitted lymph node tissue and the routine use of immunohistochemical stains, both of which had been proven, even in the pre-sentinel lymph node era, to improve detection of occult metastases, which impart a poor prognosis. While the optimal method for pathologic examination of the sentinel lymph node remains "a work in progress", examination of at least three levels of the block, and the routine use of immunohistochemical stains for antigens such as S-100 (for melanoma) and keratin proteins (for carcinoma) seems to constitute the current "standard of care". The value of highly sensitive methods, such as PCR, in the search for occult metastases remains a subject of active investigation.

REFERENCES

Albertini JJ, Lyman GH, Cox C, et al. Lymphatic mapping and sentinel node biopsy in the patient with breast cancer [see comments]. Journal of the American Medical Association 1996;276(22):1818-22

Anderson TJ. The challenge of sentinel lymph node biopsy. Histopathology 1999;35(1):82-4

Bass SS, Cox CE, Ku NN, Berman C, Reintgen DS. The role of sentinel lymph node biopsy in breast cancer. Journal of the American College of Surgeons 1999;189(2):183-94

Bieligk SC, Ghossein R, Bhattacharya S, Coit DG. Detection of tyrosinase mRNA by reverse transcription-polymerase chain reaction in melanoma sentinel nodes [see comments]. Annals of Surgical Oncology 1999;6(3):232-40

Bishop PW, Menasce LP, Yates AJ, et al. An immunophenotypic survey of malignant melanomas. Histopathology 1993;23:159-66

Black RB, Roberts MM, Stewart HJ, et al. The search for occult metastases in breast cancer: does it add to established staging methods? Australian and New Zealand Journal of Surgery 1980;50(6):574-9

Blaheta HJ, Schittek B, Breuninger H, et al. Detection of melanoma micrometastasis in sentinel nodes by reverse transcription-polymerase chain reaction correlates with tumor thickness and is predictive of micrometastatic disease in the lymph node basin. American Journal of Surgical Pathology 1999;23(7):822-8

Blessing K, Sanders DS, Grant JJ. Comparison of immunohistochemical staining of the novel antibody melan-A with S100 protein and HMB-45 in malignant melanoma and melanoma variants. Histopathology 1998;32(2):139-46

Borgstein PJ, Pijpers R, Comans EF, et al. Sentinel lymph node biopsy in breast cancer: guidelines and pitfalls of lymphoscintigraphy and gamma probe detection. Journal of the American College of Surgeons 1998;186(3):275-83

Bostick PJ, Morton DL, Turner RR, et al. Prognostic significance of occult metastases detected by sentinel lymphadenectomy and reverse transcriptase-polymerase chain reaction in early-stage melanoma patients. Journal of Clinical Oncology 1999;17(10):3238-44

Burak WE, Jr., Walker MJ, Yee LD, et al. Routine preoperative lymphoscintigraphy is not necessary prior to sentinel node biopsy for breast cancer. American Journal of Surgery 1999;177(6):445-9

Busam KJ, Chen YT, Old LJ, et al. Expression of melan-A (MART1) in benign melanocytic nevi and primary cutaneous malignant melanoma. American Journal of Surgical Pathology 1998;22(8):976-82

Cabanes PA, Salmon RJ, Vilcoq JR, et al. Value of axillary dissection in addition to lumpectomy and radiotherapy in early breast cancer. The Breast Carcinoma Collaborative Group of the Institut Curie [see comments]. Lancet 1992;339(8804):1245-8

Carter BA, Jensen RA, Simpson JF, Page DL. Benign transport of breast epithelium into axillary lymph nodes after biopsy. American Journal of Clinical Pathology 2000;113(2):259-265

Charny CK, Jacobowitz G, Melamed J, Tata M, Harris MN. Sinus histiocytosis mimicking metastatic melanoma in lymph nodes of a patient with a large joint prosthesis: case report and review of the literature. Journal of Surgical Oncology 1995;60(2):128-30

Cibull ML. Handling sentinel lymph node biopsy specimens.A work in progress. Archives of Pathology and Laboratory Medicine 1999;123(7):620-1

Clayton F, Hopkins CL. Pathologic correlates of prognosis in lymph node-positive breast carcinomas. Cancer 1993;71(5):1780-90

Cochran AJ. The pathologist's role in sentinel lymph node evaluation. Seminars in Nuclear Medicine 2000;30(1):11-7

Cochran AJ, Lu HF, Li PX, Saxton R, Wen DR. S-100 protein remains a practical marker for melanocytic and other tumours. Melanoma Research 1993;3(5):325-30

Cote RJ, Peterson HF, Chaiwun B, et al. Role of immunohistochemical detection of lymph-node metastases in management of breast cancer. International Breast Cancer Study Group. Lancet 1999;354(9182):896-900

Crossin JA, Johnson AC, Stewart PB, Turner WW, Jr. Gamma-probe-guided resection of the sentinel lymph node in breast cancer. American Surgeon 1998;64(7):666-8; discussion 669

Csemi G. Metastases in axillary sentinel lymph nodes in breast cancer as detected by intensive histopathological work up [see comments]. Journal of Clinical Pathology 1999;52(12):922-924

Czemiecki BJ, Scheff AM, Callans LS, et al. Immunohistochemistry with pancytokeratins improves the sensitivity of sentinel lymph node biopsy in patients with breast carcinoma. Cancer 1999;85(5):1098-103

Dale PS, Williams JT 4th. Axillary staging utilizing selective sentinel lymphadenectomy for patients with invasive breast carcinoma. American Surgeon 1998;64(1):28-31; discussion 32

de Mascarel I, Bonichon F, Coindre JM, Trojani M. Prognostic significance of breast cancer axillary lymph node micrometastases assessed by two special techniques: reevaluation with longer follow-up. British Journal of Cancer 1992;66(3):523-7

Domagala W, Bedner E, Chosia M, Weber K, Osborn M. Keratin-positive reticulum cells in fine needle aspirates and touch imprints of hyperplastic lymph nodes. A possible pitfall in the immunocytochemical diagnosis of metastatic carcinoma. Acta Cytologica 1992;36(2):241-5

Dowlatshahi K, Fan M, Snider HC, Habib FA. Lymph node micrometastases from breast carcinoma: reviewing the dilemma. Cancer 1997;80(7):1188-97

Fernando SS, Johnson S, Bate J. Immunohistochemical analysis of cutaneous malignant melanoma: comparison of S-100 protein, HMB-45 monoclonal antibody and NKI/C3 monoclonal antibody. Pathology 1994;26(1):16-9

Fisher ER, Palekar A, Rockette H, Redmond C, Fisher B. Pathologic findings from the National Surgical Adjuvant Breast Project (Protocol No. 4). V. Significance of axillary nodal micro- and macrometastases. Cancer 1978;42(4):2032-8

Fleming ID, Cooper JS, Henson DE, et al. AJCC Cancer Staging Manual. 5th ed. Philadelphia: Lippincott-Raven; 1997

Flett MM, Going JJ, Stanton PD, Cooke TG. Sentinel node localization in patients with breast cancer. British Journal of Surgery 1998;85(7):991-3

Foster RS. General anatomy of the lymphatic system. In: Foster RS, Cady B, editors. Surgical Oncology Clinics of North America: Lymph Nodes in Surgical Oncology. Philadelphia: WB Saunders, 1996;5(1):1-13

Frisman DM, Taylor CR. Immunohistology of the skin: melanoma, intermediate filament. In: Taylor CR, Cote RJ, editors. Immunomicroscopy: A Diagnostic Tool for the Surgical Pathologist. v 19. Philadelphia: W.B. Saunders; 1994

Gibbs JF, Huang PP, Zhang PJ, et al. Accuracy of pathologic techniques for the diagnosis of metastatic melanoma in sentinel lymph nodes. Annals of Surgical Oncology 1999;6(7):699-704

Giuliano AE, Jones RC, Brennan M, Statman R. Sentinel lymphadenectomy in breast cancer. Journal of Clinical Oncology 1997;15(6):2345-50

Giuliano AE, Kirgan DM, Guenther JM, et al. Lymphatic mapping and sentinel lymphadenectomy for breast cancer [see comments]. Annals of Surgery 1994;220:391-8; discussion 398-401

Gloghini A, Volpe R, Carbone A. Vimentin immunostaining in fibroblastic reticulum cells within human reactive and neoplastic lymphoid follicles. Human Pathology 1990;21(8):792-8

Goldhirsch A, Castiglione M. Prognostic importance of occult axillary lymph node micrometastases from breast cancers. International (Ludwig) Breast Cancer Study Group [see comments]. Lancet 1990;335:1565-8

Goscin C, Glass LF, Messina JL. Pathologic examination of the sentinel lymph node in melanoma. In: Reintgen DS, editor. Surgical Oncology Clinics of North America 1999;8(3):427-34, viii

Guenther JM, Krishnamoorthy M, Tan LR. Sentinel lymphadenectomy for breast cancer in a community managed care setting. Cancer Journal 1997;3(6):336-40

Hainsworth PJ, Tjandra JJ, Stillwell RG, et al. Detection and significance of occult metastases in node-negative breast cancer. British Journal of Surgery 1993;80(4):459-63

Hatta N, Fujimoto A, Takehara K, Takata M. Mapping of occult melanoma micrometastases in the inguinal lymph node basin by immunohistochemistry and RT-PCR. Melanoma Research 1999;9(4):401-6

Hill AD, Tran KN, Akhurst T, et al. Lessons learned from 500 cases of lymphatic mapping for breast cancer. Annals of Surgery 1999;229(4):528-35

Huvos AG, Hutter RV, Berg JW. Significance of axillary macrometastases and micrometastases in mammary cancer. Annals of Surgery 1971;173(1):44-6

Ivens D, Hoe AL, Podd TJ, et al. Assessment of morbidity from complete axillary dissection. British Journal of Cancer 1992;66(1):136-8

Jaderborg JM, Harrison PB, Kiser JL, Maynard SL. The feasibility and accuracy of the sentinel lymph node biopsy for breast carcinoma. American Surgeon 1999;65(8):699-703; discussion 704-5

Jannink I, Fan M, Nagy S, Rayudu G, Dowlatshahi K. Serial sectioning of sentinel nodes in patients with breast cancer: a pilot study [see comments]. Annals of Surgical Oncology 1998;5(4):310-4

Joseph E, Brobeil A, Cruse CW, et al. Lymphatic mapping for melanomas of the upper extremity. Journal of Hand Surgery [Am] 1999;24(4):675-81

Joseph E, Messina J, Glass FL, et al. Radioguided surgery for the ultrastaging of the patient with melanoma [see comments]. Cancer Journal 1997;3(6):341-5.

Jungbluth AA, Busam KJ, Gerald WL, et al. A103: An anti-melan-a monoclonal antibody for the detection of malignant melanoma in paraffin-embedded tissues. American Journal of Surgical Pathology 1998;22(5):595-602

Kaufmann O, Koch S, Burghardt J, Audring H, Dietel M. Tyrosinase, melan-A, and KBA62 as markers for the immunohistochemical identification of metastatic amelanotic melanomas on paraffin sections. Modern Pathology 1998;11(8):740-6

Kelemen PR, Essner R, Foshag LJ, Morton DL. Lymphatic mapping and sentinel lymphadenectomy after wide local excision of primary melanoma. Journal of the American College of Surgeons 1999;189(3):247-52

Kelley SW, Komorowski RA, Dayer AM. Axillary sentinel lymph node examination in breast carcinoma. Archives of Pathology and Laboratory Medicine 1999;123(6):533-5

Keramopoulos A, Tsionou C, Minaretzis D, Michalas S, Aravantinos D. Arm morbidity following treatment of breast cancer with total axillary dissection: a multivariated approach. Oncology 1993;50(6):445-9

Kissin MW, Querci della Rovere G, Easton D, Westbury G. Risk of lymphoedema following the treatment of breast cancer. British Journal of Surgery 1986;73(7):580-4

Koller M, Barsuk D, Zippel D, et al. Sentinel lymph node involvement--a predictor for axillary node status with breast cancer--has the time come? European Journal of Surgical Oncology 1998;24(3):166-8

Krag D. Current status of sentinel lymph node surgery for breast cancer [editorial; comment]. Journal of the National Cancer Institute 1999;91(4):302-3

Krag D, Weaver D, Ashikaga T, et al. The sentinel node in breast cancer--a multicenter validation study. New England Journal of Medicine 1998;339(14):941-6

Ku NN. Pathologic examination of sentinel lymph nodes in breast cancer. In: Reintgen DS, editor. Surgical Oncology Clinics of North America 1999;8(3):469-79

Larson D, Weinstein M, Goldberg I, et al. Edema of the arm as a function of the extent of axillary surgery in patients with stage I-II carcinoma of the breast treated with primary radiotherapy. International Journal of Radiation Oncology, Biology, Physics 1986;12(9):1575-82

Lukowsky A, Bellmann B, Ringk A, et al. Detection of melanoma micrometastases in the sentinel lymph node and in nonsentinel nodes by tyrosinase polymerase chain reaction. Journal of Investigative Dermatology 1999;113(4):554-9

McIntosh SA, Going JJ, Soukop M, Purushotham AD, Cooke TG. Therapeutic implications of the sentinel lymph node in breast cancer [letter]. Lancet 1999;354(9178):570

McMasters KM, Giuliano AE, Ross MI, et al. Sentinel-lymph-node biopsy for breast cancer--not yet the standard of care. New England Journal of Medicine 1998;339(14):990-5

Messina JL, Glass LF, Cruse CW, et al. Pathologic examination of the sentinel lymph node in malignant melanoma. American Journal of Surgical Pathology 1999;23(6):686-90

Morton DL, Chan AD. Current status of intraoperative lymphatic mapping and sentinel lymphadenectomy for melanoma: is it standard of care? Journal of the American College of Surgeons 1999;189(2):214-23

Morton DL, Wen DR, Foshag LJ, et al. Intraoperative lymphatic mapping and selective cervical lymphadenectomy for early-stage melanomas of the head and neck. Journal of Clinical Oncology 1993;11(9):1751-6

Morton DL, Wen DR, Wong JH, et al. Technical details of intraoperative lymphatic mapping for early stage melanoma. Archives of Surgery 1992;127(4):392-9

Nasser IA, Lee AK, Bosari S, et al. Occult axillary lymph node metastases in "node-negative" breast carcinoma. Human Pathology 1993;24(9):950-7

Offodile R, Hoh C, Barsky SH, et al. Minimally invasive breast carcinoma staging using lymphatic mapping with radiolabeled dextran. Cancer 1998;82(9):1704-8

O'Hea BJ, Hill AD, El-Shirbiny AM, et al. Sentinel lymph node biopsy in breast cancer: initial experience at Memorial Sloan-Kettering Cancer Center [see comments]. Journal of the American College of Surgeons 1998;186(4):423-7

Pendas S, Dauway E, Cox CE, et al. Sentinel node biopsy and cytokeratin staining for the accurate staging of 478 breast cancer patients. American Surgeon 1999;65(5):500-5; discussion 505-6

Pfeifer JD. Sentinel lymph node biopsy [editorial; comment]. American Journal of Clinical Pathology 1999;112(5):599-602

Pijpers R, Meijer S, Hoekstra OS, et al. Impact of lymphoscintigraphy on sentinel node identification with technetium-99m-colloidal albumin in breast cancer. Journal of Nuclear Medicine 1997;38(3):366-8

Reintgen D, Cruse CW, Wells K, et al. The orderly progression of melanoma nodal metastases. Annals of Surgery 1994;220(6):759-67

Rosen PP, Saigo PE, Braun DW, et al. Axillary micro- and macrometastases in breast cancer: prognostic significance of tumor size. Annals of Surgery 1981;194(5):585-91

Rubio IT, Korourian S, Cowan C, et al. Sentinel lymph node biopsy for staging breast cancer. American Journal of Surgery 1998;176(6):532-7

Schoenfeld A, Luqmani Y, Smith D, et al. Detection of breast cancer micrometastases in axillary lymph nodes by using polymerase chain reaction. Cancer Research 1994;54(11):2986-90

Schreiber RH, Pendas S, Ku NN, et al. Microstaging of breast cancer patients using cytokeratin staining of the sentinel lymph node [see comments]. Annals of Surgical Oncology 1999,6(1).95-101

Schrenk P, Rieger R, Shamiyeh A, et al. Morbidity following sentinel lymph node biopsy versus axillary node dissection for patients with breast carcinoma. Cancer 2000;88(3):608-14

Shamoto M, Hosokawa S, Shinzato M, Kaneko C. Comparison of Langerhans cells and interdigitating reticulum cells. Advances in Experimental Medicine and Biology 1993;329:311-4

Shivers SC, Wang X, Li W, et al. Molecular staging of malignant melanoma: correlation with clinical outcome. Journal of the American Medical Association 1998;280(16):1410-5

Smith PA, Harlow SP, Krag DN, et al. Submission of lymph node tissue for ancillary studies decreases the accuracy of conventional breast cancer axillary node staging. Modern Pathology 1999;12(8):781-5

Sobin LH, Wittekind C. TNM Classification of Malignant Tumours. 5th ed. New York: J. Wiley; 1997

Sudilovsky D, Cha I. Fine needle aspiration cytology of dermatopathic lymphadenitis. Acta Cytologica 1998;42(6):1341-6

Thompson JF, McCarthy WH, Bosch CM, et al. Sentinel lymph node status as an indicator of the presence of metastatic melanoma in regional lymph nodes. Melanoma Research 1995;5(4):255-60

Treseler PA, Tauchi PS. Pathologic Analysis of the Sentinel Lymph Node. In: Leong SPL, Wong JH, editors. The Surgical Clinics of North America: Sentinel Lymph Nodes in Human Solid Cancer. Philadelphia: WB Saunders, 2000;80(6):1695-1719

Turner RR, Hansen NM, Stern SL, et al. Intraoperative examination of the sentinel lymph node for breast carcinoma staging [see comments]. American Journal of Clinical Pathology 1999a;112(5):627-34

Turner RR, Ollila DW, Stern S, et al. Optimal histopathologic examination of the sentinel lymph node for breast carcinoma staging. American Journal of Surgical Pathology 1999b;23(3):263-7

Turner RR, Ollila DW, Krasne DL, et al. Histopathologic validation of the sentinel lymph node hypothesis for breast carcinoma. Annals of Surgery 1997;226(3):271-6; discussion 276-8

Van der Velde-Zimmermann D, Roijers JF, Bouwens-Rombouts A, et al. Molecular test for the detection of tumor cells in blood and sentinel nodes of melanoma patients. American Journal of Pathology 1996;149(3):759-64

Van Diest PJ. Histopathological workup of sentinel lymph nodes: how much is enough? Journal of Clinical Pathology 1999a;52(12):871-3

Van Diest PJ, Peterse HL, Borgstein PJ, Hoekstra O, Meijer CJ. Pathological investigation of sentinel lymph nodes. European Journal of Nuclear Medicine 1999b;26(4 Suppl):S43-9

Van Diest PJ, Torrenga H, Borgstein PJ, et al. Reliability of intraoperative frozen section and imprint cytological investigation of sentinel lymph nodes in breast cancer. Histopathology 1999c;35(1):14-8

Veronesi U, Paganelli G, Viale G, et al. Sentinel lymph node biopsy and axillary dissection in breast cancer: results in a large series. Journal of the National Cancer Institute 1999;91(4):368-73

Veronesi U, Paganelli G, Galimberti V, et al. Sentinel-node biopsy to avoid axillary dissection in breast cancer with clinically negative lymph-nodes [see comments]. Lancet 1997;349(9069):1864-7

Viale G, Bosari S, Mazzarol G, et al. Intraoperative examination of axillary sentinel lymph nodes in breast carcinoma patients. Cancer 1999;85(11):2433-8

Warnke RA, Weiss LM, Chan JKC, et al. Tumors of the Lymph Nodes and Spleen. 3rd ed. Washington: Armed Forces Institute of Pathology: 1995

Wells KE, Rapaport DP, Cruse CW, et al. Sentinel lymph node biopsy in melanoma of the head and neck. Plastic Reconstruction Surgery 1997;100(3):591-4

Winchester DJ, Sener SF, Winchester DP, et al. Sentinel lymphadenectomy for breast cancer: experience with 180 consecutive patients: efficacy of filtered technetium 99m sulphur colloid with overnight migration time. Journal of the American College of Surgeons 1999;188(6):597-603

Yu LL, Flotte TJ, Tanabe KK, et al. Detection of microscopic melanoma metastases in sentinel lymph nodes. Cancer 1999;86(4):617-27

6 SELECTIVE LYMPH NODE MAPPING IN COLORECTAL CANCER – A PROPSECTIVE STUDY FOR IMPACT ON STAGING, LIMITATIONS AND PITFALLS

Sukamal Saha, MD

INTRODUCTION

Colorectal cancer remains a major cause of morbidity and mortality from all gastrointestinal malignancy throughout the world, with last published account of 783,000 new cases in 1990 causing about 437,000 deaths globally [Parkin 1999]. It is the third leading cause of cancer related death in the United States with an estimated 133,200 new cases of colorectal cancer in the year 2000, causing approximately 56,500 deaths [Greenlee 2000]. The most important prognostic factor for predicting survival in colorectal cancer is the stage of the tumor during initial diagnosis. Even though surgery alone is considered curative in most patients with the disease confined within the bowel wall (AJCC stage I/II), the survival decreases significantly by about 25-35% once the disease spreads beyond the bowel wall to the draining lymph nodes (AJCC stage III). Following surgery, adjuvant chemotherapy has been shown to be curative in more than one third of patients with nodal metastasis [Woolmark 1993]. Therefore, diagnostic accuracy of nodal metastasis remains critical for proper prediction of survival and appropriate therapeutic planning. About 10-25% of patients with so-called localized disease (AJCC stage I/II) will develop progression of the disease within five years of diagnosis and die of metastatic disease in spite of having curative surgery. Even though the cause of such systemic failure may be multifactorial, it is reasonable to assume that many of these patients indeed had occult micrometastasis, which remained undetected by conventional pathologic examination. Various methods have been developed to increase the incidence of detection of such nodal micrometastasis, e.g., serial sectioning [Pickreen 1961, Turner 1999], immunohistochemistry using cytokeratin [Haboubi 1998, Greenson 1994], and most recently by reverse transcriptase polymerase chain reaction (RT-PCR) [Mori 1995]. All of these methods have indeed increased the rate of detection of nodal metastases in colorectal cancer but with an enormous burden to the pathologist in terms of time, cost and labor intensity. For these reasons, sentinel lymph node (SLN) mapping technique seems to be an ideal alternative for the accurate staging of patients with colorectal cancer.

The SLN mapping concept was originally proposed by Cabanas [1977] in 1977 for the treatment of cancer of the penis. In 1992, Morton and colleagues [Morton 1992] defined and improved the technique of SLN mapping in patients with malignant melanoma. Since the 1990's, this technique has been used for accurate staging of nodal metastasis in multiple solid tumors including breast [Giuliano 1994], head and neck, thyroid, gastrointestinal, gynecological [Bilchik 1998], lung [Little 1999], colorectal cancers [Saha 2000]. The sentinel lymph node is defined as the first to fourth node having direct drainage from the primary tumor site and has the highest potential of harboring micrometastases when present. Multiple studies [Morton 1992, Giuliano 1994] have shown the status of SLN(s) also reflect the histological features of the particular lymph node basin with more than 90% accuracy. Therefore if the SLNs can be identified during colorectal cancer surgery, these nodes can be specially tested by the pathologists for a detailed analysis by multilevel microsections, immunohistochemistry, and RT-PCR methods. This may lead to the detection of occult nodal micrometastases which would have otherwise remained undetected by conventional pathological examination of one or two sections of the lymph node. This may upstage a significant number of cases with early colorectal cancer to whom potentially curative systemic chemotherapy can then be offered which may lead to an increase in survival.

For the first time in the United States, our group has undertaken a prospective study regarding the use of SLN mapping technique in colorectal cancer. The purpose of the study is five-fold: 1) to determine the feasibility of SLN mapping using isosulfan blue dye (Lymphazurin 1%, Ben Venue Labs, Inc., Bedford, Ohio, USA; 2) to assess the accuracy of the SLNs in determining the status of regional nodes; 3) to identify any aberrant mesenteric lymphatic drainage patterns; 4) to assess the limitations and pitfalls of the technique in patients with colorectal cancer; and 5) to evaluate the use of any other dye for the mapping technique.

SELECTIVE SENTINEL LYMPH NODE MAPPING FOR COLON CANCER: HOW WE DO IT

From October 1996 through January 2000, 159 consecutive patients with the diagnosis of colorectal cancers were prospectively studied under an Institutional Review Committee approved protocol after informed consent was obtained. Preoperative evaluation for all patients included a complete history and physical examination, routine laboratory studies, including liver function study and carcinoembryonic antigen (CEA), colonoscopy, and computed tomography of the abdomen and pelvis. Prior to surgery all patients were given standard bowel prep along with oral and intravenous antibiotics. In all patients, the surgeon had a prior knowledge (by the colonoscopy procedure) of the approximate location of the primary tumor. An exploratory laparotomy was performed to find the extent of the primary tumor and any distant metastases. Some mobilization of the bowel along the paracolic gutter was needed to deliver the bowel adjoining the tumor near the surface. Mesenteric dissection was kept at a minimum to prevent disruption of the lymphatic pathway.

Injection of Lymphazurin

Once the tumor bearing area of the colon was isolated, 1-2 ml. of Lymphazurin 1% was injected subserosally by a tuberculin syringe around the primary tumor in a circumferential manner (Figure 1). Care was taken not to inject into the lumen of the bowel. For low rectal lesions the dye was injected by a 27-gauge spinal needle through a proctoscope, into the submucosal and muscular layer underneath the tumor.

Identification of Lymphatic Basins

The blue dye travels quickly via the lymphatics to the draining lymph nodes, which turn pale to deep blue. The first to fourth blue nodes closest to the tumor with the most direct drainage from the tumor are marked as "SLN(s)". The SLN(s) are usually identified within the first five to seven minutes following the injection. They are usually seen on the retro peritoneal surface and marked with suture for future identification (Figure 2). Once the SLNs are identified, a standard oncologic resection is then performed to include adequate proximal and distal margins, along with the regional lymph nodes in the attached mesentery. Occasionally a blue nodeis identified outside of the usual lymphatic bearing area and should be considered as an SLN and included within the margins of the resection. Occasionally, in patients with unusually thick or fatty mesentery, limited surgical dissection of the mesenteric fat was required to identify the blue-stained lymph nodes.

Due to the recent reports of rare anaphylactic reactions to the Lymphazurin dye [Leong 2000] attempts are being made to validate the use of other dyes for SLN mapping technique. For this purpose, we also used a commonly used dye, Fluorescein 10%, 1-2 ml mixed with Lymphazurin. Fluorescein dye also was found to travel via the lymphatics to nearby SLN(s), and turned the blue sentinel node to greenish-yellow in color (Figure 3). This was further confirmed by Wood's light illumination in a darkened room as fluorescent bright yellow nodes. No allergic reaction has been observed during the use of either Lymphazurin or Fluorescein dye in our series.

PATHOLOGICAL EXAMINATION

The surgical specimens were sent to the pathology lab in a fresh state. The SLNs were dissected free from the specimen and sectioned grossly at about 2-3 mm. intervals and blocked separately in individual cassettes; the entire specimen must be examined for proper evaluation of the tumor and harvesting of nonSLNs. The pericolic adipose tissues were often fixed for 2 to 18 hours in Carnoy's fluid [Wiese 2000] to aid in the recognition and dissection of additional nonSLNs. For each SLN, usually a total of 10 sections were cut through the blocks at a thickness of 4 microns, each approximately 20-40 microns apart. One of these sections, usually at the 5th level, was immunostained for the demonstration of low molecular weight cytokeratin (AE-1 and AE-3 cocktail; Ventana, Tucson, AZ) (Figure 4). The other sections were stained routinely with hematoxylin and eosin (H&E). A small sample of the SLN along with a piece of a nonSLN and the primary tumor were sent to a central laboratory for RT-PCR study.

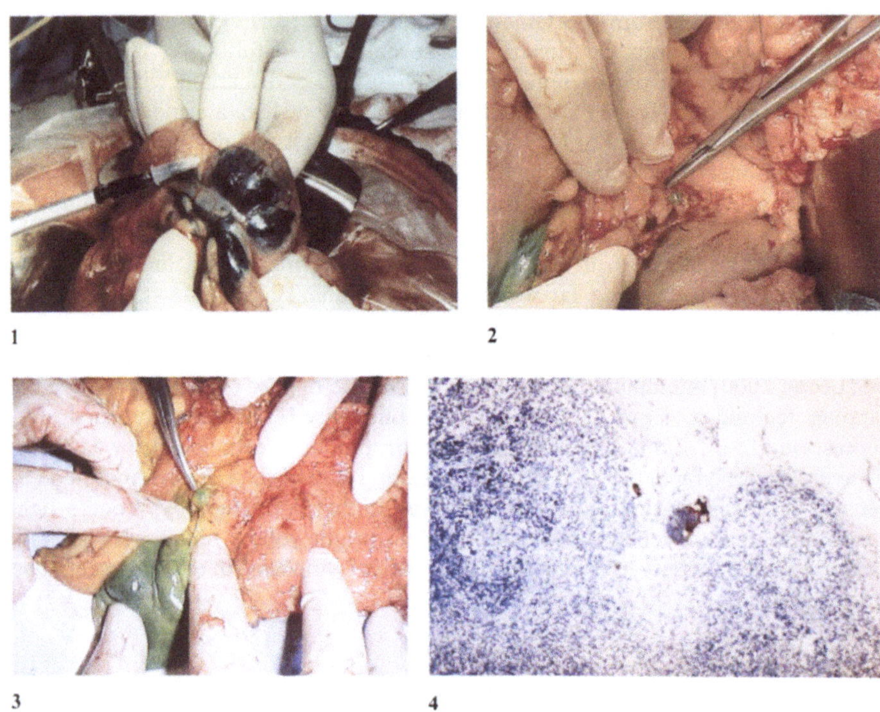

Figure 1. Lymphazurin 1% is being injected subserosally around a tumor in the sigmoid colon of a 70-year old female.
Figure 2. The sentinel lymph node is marked with suture as they appear soon after the dye injection.
Figure 3. Fluorescein 10% is also being injected subserosally showing greenish- yellow stained sentinel lymph node near the primary tumor.
Figure 4.   Occult micrometastasis seen in a small 9 mm sentinel lymph node detected only by immunohistochemistry.

CLINICAL OUTCOME

Of the 159 consecutive patients in this study, 93 had colon, 41 rectosigmoid and 25 had rectal cancer. The number and locations of the primary tumors were as follows: cecum 31; right colon 41; transverse colon 15; splenic flexure 2; left colon 4; sigmoid colon 26; rectosigmoid colon 15; and rectum 25 respectively. Ages ranged from 33-97 years (median 71 years). The SLN mapping technique successfully identified 1-4 SLNs in 156 out of 159 patients (98%). In three patients, the SLN mapping technique failed to identify any blue node (2 with rectal cancer treated with neoadjuvant chemo/radiation therapy and one with perforated colon cancer). The following analysis is based on the remaining 156 patients in whom at least one SLN was identified. A total of 2,425 lymph nodes were examined (mean 15.5 per patient), of which 286 (12%) lymph nodes were identified as SLNs. Of these, one SLN was identified in 40% pts, two SLNs in 40% pts, three SLNs in 18% pts and four SLNs in 2% pt. In 98 (63%) patients the SLNs were negative for metastasis. Of these 98 patients, 91 (93%) patients the SLNs, as well as all the nonSLNs were negative for metastasis. In the other seven (4%) patients, the SLNs were negative but eleven of the nonSLNs were positive for metastasis (skip metastasis). In 58 patients, the SLNs were positive for metastasis; of these, in 31 patients, the SLNs were the only site of metastasis with all other nonSLNs being negative. In 23 (15% of the total 156 patients) of these patients, micrometastasis were identified only in 1-2 of ten microsections of a single SLN. Of these 23, ten (6.4%) were confirmed by immunohistochemistry only; thus representing true occult micrometastasis. The extent of surgery was altered by evidence of an aberrant lymphatic pathway detected by the SLN mapping technique in seven patients. Overall, the sensitivity of SLN mapping for colorectal cancer in our series was 93.7%; specificity of 100%; and negative predictive value of 93%. Solitary metastasis in one SLN, as was found in 15% of patients, may have upstaged these patients from AJCC stage I/II to stage III, who may then benefit from adjuvant chemotherapy.

Incidence of metastasis in SLNs vs nonSLNs 26% vs 9.5% respectively. In presence of negative SLNs metastasis were found in 12 out of 2,139 (0.6%) of nonSLNs only (skip metastasis). To evaluate the effect of multilevel micro sectioning of the SLNs only as opposed to the nonSLNs, for the first 25 consecutive patients all SLNs as well as the nonSLNs were sectioned at 10 levels in identical manner. Of the 390 lymph nodes examined (average 15.6 per patient), 13 (36%) of the 36 SLNs were positive for metastasis, while only 24 (7%) of the 354 nonSLNs had metastasis. When all the initially negative nonSLNs were sectioned at 10 levels and reexamined, only 0.6% (2 of 330 lymph nodes) revealed previously undetected micrometastasis. These results further confirm the unique distribution of metastasis via the lymphatics to the SLNs with minimal chance of skip metastasis. Thus, there may be no further benefit in performing multilevel sections of the nonSLNs as opposed to the SLNs.

OVERVIEW

Lymph node metastasis decreases the overall survival in most solid tumors as in breast, melanoma, and colorectal cancer by about 30%. For colorectal cancer with lymph node metastasis, adjuvant chemotherapy is the recommended treatment, with a reduction in cancer-related mortality by approximately 33% [Cohen 1998]. The ability to detect micrometastasis in SLNs may upstage patients from AJCC stage I/II to stage III, thereby altering the post surgical treatment plan to include adjuvant chemotherapy. This study confirms that in patients with colorectal cancer, as in breast and melanoma, SLN mapping technique is highly successful (98%) and accurate (96%). The failure to identify SLNs in two patients with preoperative chemo/radiation therapy for low rectal cancer may be due to submucosal fibrosis caused by the radiation therapy. The other patient with perforated carcinoma had intense peritoneal reaction, thereby preventing the dye from entering into the enlarged, inflamed lymph nodes. Of the seven patients with skip metastasis in this series, two had two closely situated primary tumors; two patients had large T4 tumors of rectosigmoid invading adjacent organs; one patient had previous colectomy with anastomotic recurrence. Potential limitations and contraindications of this procedure are shown in Table 1.

TABLE 1

Limitations and Contra-indications of Sentinel Lymph Node Mapping

Limitations
Previous colon surgery
Neoadjuvant chemo/radiation therapy
Large tumor invading adjacent organs
Perforated carcinoma
Multiple primary tumors

Contra-indications
Distant metastasis
Clinically positive lymph nodes

This study also confirms that in colorectal cancer patient, SLN mapping is technically simple with a short learning curve. Use of Fluorescein dye in the last 40 patients also allowed us to further validate the lymphatic mapping technique by the use of Wood's light illumination in a darkened room. In patients with thick mesentery where blue lymphatic channel is difficult to visualize, as well as in patients who may be allergic to Lymphazurin, Fluorescein dye may be an alternative for lymphatic mapping in colorectal cancer. These dyes have been found to have no apparent side effects in our series; the technique usually takes less than ten minutes of operating time; and it is relatively inexpensive ($99/vial of Lymphazurin and $5/vial of Fluorescein). Unlike in melanoma and breast cancer, no radionuclide dye or gamma probe was used in this study thereby further reducing the cost.

It should be noted that failure to inject the dye completely circumferentially, as well as injection of the dye into the lumen, might lead to skip metastasis. Hence, every attempt should be made to inject the dye subserosally to prevent intraluminal injection and to inject at multiple points surrounding the tumor. Utmost precaution should be taken not to spill the dye, especially the Fluorescein, outside the bowel, which may stain non-tumor bearing areas, thereby preventing the identification of the blue lymph nodes.

SLN mapping also allows the pathologist to meticulously examine only 1-4 SLNs, thereby increasing the chance of diagnosis of micrometastasis. Multilevel microsections of the SLNs only may allow us to accurately predict the nodal status with a very low incidence of skip metastasis. This may allow the pathologist to avoid costly and time-consuming examination of the large number of the nonSLNs with multilevel microsections. Immunohistochemistry and PCR technique may further enhance the diagnosis of nodal micrometastasis.

A large, multi-institutional study is being proposed by the American College of Surgeons Oncology Group (ACOSOG - Z0170) to evaluate and to verify the efficacy of this technique and to assess its impact on the survival of patients with colorectal cancer. It is our hope that the application of SLN mapping technique in colorectal cancer will become part of the standard practice of the general surgeons given its simplicity, high accuracy, low cost, and its ability to aid the pathologists to focus their attention on 1-4 SLNs for detailed analysis, thereby upstaging a significant number of patients. Thus upstaged, patients may be offered newer adjuvant chemotherapy, which may alter their survival.

REFERENCES

Bilchik A, Giuliano A, Essner R, et al. Universal application of intraoperative lymphatic mapping and sentinel lymphadenectomy in solid neoplasms. Cancer Journal 1998;4(6):351-358

Cabanas RM. An approach for treatment of penile carcinoma. Cancer 1977;39(2):456-6

Cohen AM, Kelsen D, Saltz L, et al. Adjuvant therapy for colorectal cancer. Curr Prob Cancer 1998;22:5-65

Greenlee RT, Murray T, Bolden S, Wingo PA. Cancer Statistics, 2000. CA: A Cancer Journal for Clinicians 2000;50(1):7-33

Greenson JK, Isenhart CE, Rice R, et al. Identification of occult micrometastases in pericolic lymph nodes of Dukes' B colorectal cancer patients using monoclonal antibodies against cytokeratin and CC49; correlation with long-term survival. Cancer 1994;73(3):563-9

Giuliano AE, Kirgan DM, Guenther JM, Morton DL. Lymphatic mapping and sentinel lymphadenectomy for breast cancer. Annals of Surgery 1994;220(3):391-401

Haboubi NY, Abdalla SA, Amini S, et al. The novel combination of fat clearance and immunohistochemistry improves prediction of the outcome of patients with colorectal carcinomas: a preliminary study. International Journal of Colorectal Disease 1998;13(2):99-102

Leong SPL, Donegan E, Heffernon W, et al. Adverse reactions to isosulfan blue during selective sentinel lymph node dissection in melanoma. Annals of Surgical Oncology 2000;7(5):361-366

Little AG, DeHoyos A, Kirgan DM, et al. Intraoperative lymphatic mapping for non-small cell lung cancer: the sentinel node technique. Journal of Thoracic and Cardiovascular Surgery 1999;117(2):220-34

Mori M, Mimori K, Inoue H, et al. Detection of cancer micrometastases in lymph nodes by reverse transcriptase polymerase chain reaction. Cancer Research 1995;55(25):3417-20

Morton, DL, Wen DR, Wong HH, et al. Technical details of intraoperative lymphatic mapping for early stage melanoma. Archives of Surgery 1992;127(4):392-9

Parkin DM, Pisani P, Ferlay J. Global Cancer Statistics. CA: A Cancer Journal for Clinicians 1999;49(1):33-64

Pickreen JW. Significance of occult metastases, a study of breast cancer. Cancer 1961;14:1261-1271

Saha S, Wiese D, Badin J, et al. Technical details of sentinel lymph node mapping in colorectal cancer and its impact on staging. Annals of Surgical Oncology, 2000;7(2):120-124

Turner RR, Ollila DW, Stern S, Giuliano AE. Optimal histopathologic examination of the sentinel lymph node for breast carcinoma staging. American Journal of Surgical Pathology 1999;23(3):263-7

Wiese D, Saha S, Badin J. Pathologic evaluation of sentinel lymph nodes in colorectal carcinoma. Arch Pathol Lab Med 2000;124:1759-1763

Wolmark N, Rockette H, Fisher B, et al. The benefit of leucovorin-modulated fluorouracil as postoperative adjuvant therapy for primary colon cancer: Results from National Surgical Adjuvant Breast and Bowel Project protocol C-03. Journal of Clinical Oncology 1993;11(10):1879-1887

SELECTED READINGS

Haagensen CD, Feind CR, Herter FP, et al. The Lymphatics in Cancer; W. B. Saunders; 1972.

Cochran AJ, Balda BR, Starz H, et al. The Augsburg Consensus: Techniques of Lymphatic Mapping, Sentinel Lymphadenectomy, and Completion Lymphadenectomy in Cutaneous Malignancies. Cancer 2000;89(2):236-241

Eshima D, Fauconnier T, Eshima L, Thornback JR. Radiopharmaceuticals for Lymphoscintigraphy: Including Dosimetry and Radiation Considerations. Seminars in Nuclear Medicine 2000;30:25-32

Haigh PI, Giuliano AE. Operative Techniques in General Surgery: Surgical Management of Benign and Malignant Breast Disease. Philadelphia; W. B. Saunders; 2000.

Kapteijn BAE. Biopsy of the Sentinel Node in Melanoma, Penile Carcinoma and Breast Carcinoma: The case for lymphatic mapping. Amsterdam: PrintPartners Ipskamp; 1997.

Keshtgar MRS, Waddington WA, Lakhani SR, Ell PJ. The Sentinel Node in Surgical Oncology. New York: Springer; 1999.

Leong SPL, Wong JH, editors. Surgical Clinics of North America: Sentinel Lymph Nodes in Human Solid Cancer. Philadelphia: WB Saunders, 2000;80(6).

Nieweg OE, Essner R, Reintgen DS, Thompson JF, editors. Lymphatic Mapping and Probe Applications in Oncology. New York: Marcel Dekker; 2000.

Schlag PM, Veronesi U, editors. Recent Results in Cancer Research: Lymphatic Metastasis and Sentinel Lymphonodectomy. Berlin: Springer-Verlag; 2000.

Uren RF, Thompson JF, Howman-Giles RB. Lymphatic Drainage of the Skin and Breast: Locating the Sentinel Nodes. Singapore: Harwood Academic Publishers; 1999.

Whitman ED, Reintgen D. Radioguided Surgery. Austin: Landes Bioscience; 1999.

A

Allis clamp, 45, 49, 56, 59, 60
Army and Navy, 45

B

Baily right angle, 45, 59
Breast Cancer, 4, 5, 9, 14, 17, 20, 21, 33,
    65, 66, 67, 69, 72, 73, 74, 75, 81, 82,
    83, 84, 85, 86, 87, 88, 89, 90, 91, 95,
    96, 97, 98, 101
Breslow thickness, 46, 51, 52, 53, 58

C

Carcinoma, 2, 9, 65, 70, 71, 72, 84, 86,
    87, 88, 89, 91, 93, 94, 95, 97, 99, 100,
    101, 103, 114
Chemotherapy
    adjuvant, 109, 113, 114, 115
Collimator, 15, 18, 19, 20, 21, 27, 60, 69
    pinhole, 19, 27, 69
Colon Cancer, 110, 113, 116

D

Deaver retractor, 45, 49
Dye
blue, 3, 9, 16, 17, 22, 25, 40, 41, 42, 43,
    44, 46, 50, 51, 52, 53, 56, 60, 61, 65,
    66, 67, 68, 70, 71, 72, 75, 76, 110, 111
    Fluorescein, 111, 112, 114, 115
    isosulfan blue, 3, 4, 40, 50, 51, 52, 53,
    54, 55, 56, 65, 70, 75

E

Erythema, 50

G

Gamma camera, 19, 24, 42, 69
Gamma probe, 4, 19, 20, 21, 22, 25, 34,
    40, 41, 42, 43, 44, 45, 46, 51, 52, 53,
    54, 56, 60, 61, 69, 70, 75, 76, 114

    hand-held, 38, 40, 42, 43, 44, 46, 61,
    70, 76,

I

Injection
    intradermal, 3, 11, 14, 16, 17, 18, 29,
    30, 50, 51, 53, 54, 66, 67, 69, 70, 72
    parenchymal, 10, 14, 15, 16, 17, 18,
    29, 32, 33
    peritumoral, 17, 66, 67, 68, 69, 70

L

Lidocaine, 11, 13
Lumpectomy, 66, 71, 72, 76
Lymph node
    radiolabeled, 40, 44,
    regional, 2, 3, 40, 47, 59, 65, 73, 81,
    82, 83, 85, 111
Lymph node dissection, 1, 9, 39, 40, 48,
    50, 53, 54, 56, 58, 59, 60, 66, 70, 71,
    72, 73, 81, 83, 86
    axillary, 66, 70, 72, 73
    elective lymph node dissection
    (ELND), 39, 59
Lymphadenectomy, 1, 2, 3, 4, 5, 6, 9, 45,
    46, 50, 57, 58, 59, 65, 73, 74, 75, 95
    sentinel, 5, 9, 39, 45, 46, 49, 50, 57,
    59, 61, 65, 73, 74, 75, 76, 77
Lymphangiography, 9
Lymphatic
    channel, 3, 4, 9, 11, 14, 19, 22, 23, 28,
    30, 42, 43, 46, 47, 66, 67, 75, 114
    drainage, 2, 3, 4, 10, 45, 67, 82, 110
Lymphazurin, 40, 41, 43, 56, 57, 70, 71,
    110, 111, 112, 114

M

Macrophage, 9
Mapping,
    intraoperative, 40, 41, 42, 43, 50, 51,
    58, 59, 70, 72
    intraoperative lymphatic, 2, 3, 4, 50,
    52, 53, 54, 65, 70, 72, 74
Masking, 31, 32
Mastectomy, 66,
McBurney, 45, 49
Melanoma,
    cutaneous, 1, 3, 4, 5
    malignant, 9, 39, 48, 52, 56, 58, 98,
    110

Metastases, 1, 2, 4, 39, 72, 81, 82, 83, 84,
85, 86, 87, 88, 91, 93, 94, 95, 96, 98,
99, 101, 102, 103, 109, 110
nodal, 1, 39, 81, 82, 86, 87, 88, 95, 109
occult, 85, 86, 87, 91, 99, 103
regional nodal, 1, 81, 82, 95
Metastatic,
disease, 1, 2, 5, 56, 59, 71, 73, 101,
102, 109
tumor, 4, 81, 83, 85, 88, 95, 97, 103
Micrometastatic disease, 1

N

Node dissection, 1, 2, 3, 4, 5, 6, 7, 9, 33,
39, 40, 48, 50, 53, 54, 56, 58, 59, 60,
65, 66, 70, 71, 72, 73, 74, 81, 82, 83,
85, 86, 95
Node negative, 2, 5

P

Palpable mass, 14
Persistence oscilloscope (P-Scope), 19,
22, 23
Polymerase chain reaction (PCR), 101,
102, 103, 109, 110, 112, 115

R

Radiocolloid, 2, 9, 11, 13, 14, 15, 16, 17,
18, 23, 40, 41, 42, 44, 46, 50, 61, 69,
70
Radioisotope, 40, 41, 42, 43, 44, 60
Radiotracers, 9, 66

S

Shine through effect, 18, 60, 66, 69
Stain,
H&E, 84, 85, 86, 88, 87, 89, 90, 91,
95, 98, 99, 101
immunohistochemical, 57, 65, 86, 87,
88, 91, 92, 94, 101, 102, 103
immunoperoxidase, 86, 90, 91, 92, 93,
94, 96, 97, 98, 99, 101
keratin, 87, 88, 99
Sulfur colloid, 4, 10, 11, 13, 14, 16, 32,
34, 40, 42, 56, 69, 71, 75
Sentinel lymph node (SLN), 1, 3, 4, 5, 9,
12, 17, 20, 21, 25, 29, 31, 34, 39, 41,
42, 47, 48, 50, 51, 52, 53, 56, 65, 69,
71, 72, 81, 82, 83, 84, 85, 86, 87, 88,
89, 90, 91, 92, 93, 94, 95, 96, 97, 98,
99, 100, 101, 102, 103, 110, 112, 114,
115

T

Technetium 99m (Tc99m), 10, 11, 14,
16, 18, 19, 22, 23, 32, 34, 40, 41, 42,
69, 75
albumin, 10, 11, 40

U

Urticaria, 43, 50

V

Vein retractor, 45

W

Wheal, 11, 12, 23, 75

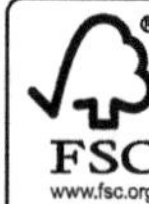

MIX
Papier aus verantwortungsvollen Quellen
Paper from responsible sources
FSC® C105338

If you have any concerns about our products,
you can contact us on
ProductSafety@springernature.com

In case Publisher is established outside the EU,
the EU authorized representative is:
Springer Nature Customer Service Center GmbH
Europaplatz 3, 69115 Heidelberg, Germany

Printed by Libri Plureos GmbH
in Hamburg, Germany